AF552391

Miracles on Park Avenue

MIRACLES
on Park Avenue

by

Albert B. Gerber

Lyle Stuart Inc. ***Secaucus, New Jersey***

This book was not authorized by Dr. Milton Reder.

Published by Lyle Stuart Inc.
120 Enterprise Ave., Secaucus, N.J. 07094
In Canada: Musson Book Company
A division of General Publishing Co. Limited.
Don Mills, Ontario

Queries regarding rights and permissions should be addressed to: Lyle Stuart, 120 Enterprise Avenue, Secaucus, N.J. 07094

Manufactured in the United States of America

Library of Congress Cataloging-in-Publication Data

Gerber, Albert Benjamin, 1913–
Miracles on Park Avenue.

Bibliography: p.
1. Pterygopalatine ganglion—Effect of drugs on.
2. Nerve block. 3. Cocaine—Physiological effect.
4. Pain—Treatment. 5. Reder, Milton. 6. Physicians—
New York (City)—Biography. I. Title.
RD84.G47 1986 615′.7822 85-27665
ISBN 0-8184-0387-X

To Jenny, J. J., Sarah,
Hank and Matthew

CONTENTS

INTRODUCTION

Why and How I Researched This Book

It all started when I began to have trouble playing tennis. All my life I have been physically active, enjoying participation in competitive sports. I spent many years playing handball several times a week. In between, I played tennis and volleyball as time permitted. In fact, ever since I was a child I could be found every day on one court or another, and many times on more than one court on the same day.

Then I noticed that I just didn't get around the court as fast as I had been able to. My legs simply stopped following orders. Finally, even when I did my exercises, they objected by giving me real pain.

The symptoms were clearly those of claudication, so my physician sent me for assorted tests. These showed no impairment of circulation, but the pain continued. I reached the stage where I couldn't walk one city block without pain.

One day one of my tennis partners heard David Brenner on the Regis Philbin Cable Health News television program. Brenner spoke glowingly about a Dr. Milton Reder of New York, who had treated him for a variety of pains in lower back, legs and elsewhere.

I had no problem getting Dr. Reder's address and phone number, and I phoned to make an appointment. (I learned later that no appointment is necessary. If the office was open, Dr. Reder saw patients on a first-come basis.)

I walked into the office at 555 Park Avenue, anticipating a standard doctor's waiting room. My eyes would not believe what they saw! Fifteen people of both sexes were scattered around a large room in various states of repose, some reading, some reclining, some just sitting and staring into space, but all with one startling similarity—they had what appeared to be wires with knobs on the end extending from their noses!

I carried a large manila folder in which were my x-rays and other medical reports. When it was my turn to see Dr. Reder, I presented my folder. He looked through it with interest. I learned later that he had not expected such a presentation. Most of his patients arrive empty-handed, simply telling him they have a pain here or there and asking him to please make it go away.

The then-current diagnosis for my condition was "spinal stenosis" (the spine narrowing and impinging on the nerves running down both legs). I asked Dr. Reder if his treatment could help such a condition. I received what I later learned was his stock reply.

He smiled and said, "I can't be sure. Sometimes it works for a stenosis, and sometimes it doesn't. All we can do is give it a try."

He questioned me about allergies, medications, and a few other possibly pertinent aspects of my general health. After a few minutes he was ready to insert what are called the applicators. He assured me that I would feel no pain. He handed me a tissue (he does this with all his patients), telling me I might shed an involuntary tear or two, since the applicators upon insertion pass by the tear ducts. I felt absolutely nothing. I did not tear, and the applicators passed through my nostrils and up to the ganglion with ease and with barely any sensation. Once they were inserted, I felt nothing.

When my treatment was completed, I circulated around the waiting area, talking to other patients. I learned very quickly that a single treatment was far from a cure. It often would take five to ten and sometimes even twenty treatments before an individual attained the desired relief. Like so many who come to Dr. Reder, I was desperate for relief. Since I live in Philadelphia, I opted to remain in New York for a few days to begin a course of treatments. I returned regularly twice a day for a period of time, and then switched to long week-ends.

I disliked just sitting around, but it was a necessary part of the regimen. I whiled away time by talking to the other patients in the office. Their stories astonished me.

Excited by what I was hearing, I called my publisher, Lyle Stuart, and told him where I was and what I was learning. I suggested that he would find it an interesting experience to visit Dr. Reder's office with me. I really had no thought at that time of writing a book about it, but I wanted to share my observations.

Lyle, intrigued by what I had to say, made an appointment to meet me at Penn Station one morning, when I came in from Philadelphia for my regular visit. He went with me to Dr. Reder's Park Avenue office to see for himself what went on.

As he spoke to the patients, Lyle quickly became enthusiastic over what he saw and heard. Some of the people knew Lyle both from the books he published and the books he wrote, and talked quite openly with him. He recognized very quickly the possibility of a book on the subject of Dr.

Milton Reder and the "sphenopalatine ganglion blockade." I had considered writing an article for *The New Yorker* or *New York* magazine. I had thought of contacting "60 Minutes" about it. But a book had not entered my mind.

But Lyle, with the publisher's eye, knew a book when he saw one. He said, "Al, I think there's a very exciting story here. I want you to get to work on it immediately!"

The only other time I had ever seen Lyle so excited about my doing a book for him was when he wanted me to write a biography of Howard Hughes (which, incidentally, I did).

That book, *Bashful Billionaire,* made *The New York Times* best-seller list and proved the correctness of Lyle Stuart's judgment. So, I thought to myself, if Lyle thinks it would make an interesting book, I'll give it a try.

In the beginning, I thought I would get a release from every patient with whom I spoke. I dutifully prepared the proper legal document (no big trick for me after being a Philadelphia lawyer for almost fifty years) and I continued my visits to Dr. Reder, both for treatment and to interview the patients, with Dr. Reder's blessings.

I discovered very quickly that most of the patients did not want to speak for publication if it meant using their own names in the book. Some people agreed to sign releases, but then the interviews with them were vague. Others simply flatly refused to sign a release at all. What I heard was, "I'll tell you my story, but you can't use my name." This held true especially for physicians, dentists, and other professional people. They seemed to feel that their use of the treatment could be construed as a reflection on their professional standing.

Faced with so many refusals to be directly quoted or identified, I abandoned the idea of using real names. Thus the names and occupations used in this book, with a few exceptions, are fictitious. Nevertheless, the stories are accurate and true. When I speak of someone like David Brenner, I use his real name, because he spoke on the record and registered no objection to the use of his name. Also, following an age-old legal precept that holds it is hard to invade the privacy of a deceased person, I do use the names of those famous patients of Dr. Reder who have died. Some cases are clear cut. One case in point: Tallulah Bankhead refers to Dr. Reder in her best-selling autobiography, *Tallulah,* making it clear in the book that her visits to him were not secret.

Miracles on Park Avenue

CHAPTER I

In Which I See a Miracle

Joyce Jarman is a pretty girl. Perhaps not pretty enough to win a beauty contest, but certainly attractive enough to command a man's attention in almost any setting. She is well-built, clear skinned and healthy-looking. However, her body is bent over and her left leg is stiffly extended.

Joyce enters Dr. Milton Reder's inner office with diffidence and a hint of trepidation. This is normal because the first sight of the office is unsteadying. The party atmosphere is fostered by large numbers of people wandering about or seated or lounging in various postures, either alone or deep in conversation with others. The bizarre effect results from wires extending from their noses. Unlike any other doctor's office I've been in, Dr. Reder's treatment room is open on two sides so that people can wander in and out at will. Informality is the order of the day.

Because Joyce is a new patient, the receptionist leads her to the doorway and introduces her to Dr. Reder, saying simply, "Doctor, this is a new patient."

The words "new patient" act as a signal to most of those who are seated or standing in the doctor's inner office. They migrate to the outer lounge, because Dr. Reder has made it well known that he wants his first interview with a new patient to be private and confidential.

The octogenarian Dr. Reder smiles warmly and reassuringly at Joyce and invites her to sit in front of him. He begins his series of standard questions:

"Are you currently taking any medication?" The answer is negative.

"Are you now, or have you recently been, on any drugs of any nature?" Joyce shakes her head again.

"Do you have any allergies?" Again the answer is "No."

The questioning continues until the doctor is assured that Joyce is a good candidate for his treatment.

He asks, "What pain killers do you take?"

She replies, "Only Tylenol, because some of the others make me sick. But I haven't had any Tylenol today."

Dr. Reder nods approvingly and continues his questioning. "I'm sure you've been to see other doctors, haven't you?" She replies, "Yes."

He asks, "What diagnosis did they give you?"

She answers, "They tell me I have a disc of my vertebra which is pressing against my sciatic nerve. It causes severe pain down my leg. I can hardly straighten my leg or step on it. I had to literally drag myself to get here."

The doctor says, "All right, we'll give this a try and see if it does you any good. I'm going to insert applicators wrapped with medicated cotton into your nose. As they pass a certain point, your eyes may tear. This is natural, so don't worry about it. You won't have any pain from the applicator, and it won't cause you discomfort."

He then takes a thin wire applicator about six inches long with a knob at one end and wraps absorbent cotton around the other end. When he has four applicators securely wrapped, he dips one of them into a small brown bottle, which contains a solution of from 10 percent to 25 percent cocaine, depending on his decision with respect to the individual patient. (Most patients receive the 25 percent solution, but he may use a weaker one in the early stages of treatment.)

With the consummate skill that comes from performing a procedure thousands of times, Dr. Reder gently inserts the first of the four applicators into the nostrils of Joyce Jarman. He wiggles the applicator so that it will pass through various apertures until it reaches a small button called a ganglion. This process is the famed sphenopalatine ganglion blockade, words the habitues of the Reder ménage toss around with easy abandon, but which take most patients two or three visits to learn to pronounce.

After he inserts one applicator into the right nostril, he inserts one into the left nostril. These are followed by a second into the right, and a second into the left. In most cases, the entire procedure takes about two minutes. With this part of the treatment finished, he tries to get Joyce Jarman to relax.

He tells her, "You aren't going to feel any results immediately, so just relax and don't worry about anything."

Joyce has already observed that many patients walk around or sit in another room, so she rises to follow the pattern. However, stretching out a shaky hand, Dr. Reder stops her. "No, I want you to sit here for a while." (He does this with all new patients. He likes to observe them, and at some point may explain that occasionally a patient has an unusual reaction, but that in almost every instance it is psychosomatic rather than physical. Nevertheless, the reaction may occur, and he wants the patient to be within his view.)

Joyce Jarman sits and visibly becomes more at ease with the strange apparatus in her nostrils. She gradually relaxes.

Other patients come in for their insertions, or removals. He uses another chair alongside Joyce's, and performs the procedure on them. Life in Doctor Reder's inner sanctum continues at a normal pace.

Approximately fifteen minutes pass. Joyce says diffidently, "You know, Dr. Reder, I think the pain is going. I would like to try to straighten out my leg. Is it all right?"

Dr. Reder smiles warmly. "Of course. That's what's supposed to happen. Straighten out your leg. Try anything you want. I'll watch you."

Joyce slowly and timorously straightens her left leg, which has been continually bent. A pleased smile crosses her face. She remarks to the interested observers, "I haven't been able to straighten that leg without pain for months."

Having straightened out the leg, a look of determination replaces the smile. "I think I would like to stand up. Is that all right?"

Dr. Reder replies, "Young lady, you can stand up, or jog around the waiting room if you want to."

Slowly, and with obviously mounting excitement, Joyce Jarman rises to her feet. Still not trusting her new-found freedom from pain, she holds on to a chair alongside of her, and takes a tentative step. She smiles triumphantly, "And I didn't feel any pain!"

Joyce takes a few careful steps, smiling broadly, and then turns to face the watching doctor. "Dr. Reder, I'm wearing an orthopedic belt . . . " She pulls up her sweater and shows the bulky orthopedic garment she is wearing under it. "I've been wearing this darn thing almost continuously for six months. I would love to take it off. Would that be all right?"

Dr. Reder nods. "Take off anything you want to take off. You won't feel any pain."

To the ripping sound of velcro separating, she triumphantly pulls off the belt and stands looking around. She nods with satisfaction. "It's a miracle!" she exclaims.

CHAPTER II

What It Is

The sphenopalatine ganglion blockade is nothing new. In fact, it goes back to 1909, to Greenfield Sluder. Dr. Sluder was a professor and Director of the Department of Otolaryngology at Washington University School of Medicine in St. Louis. The medical dictionary definition of this type of specialist is, "One skilled in the practice of otology, rhinology, and laryngology." In short, an ear, nose and throat specialist.

Dr. Sluder was looking for some form of therapy for treatment of head pains such as cluster headaches and migraine variants. As he studied anatomy, he concluded that the little ganglion situated in the head just above the top of the nose, was an important pathway for the pain. Sluder's early treatments concentrated on the destruction of the ganglion, reasoning that if he could block the pathway, he could relieve the pain. He used alcohol to do this, in some cases injecting it into the ganglion through the cheek instead of going through the nasal passage. It worked.

In 1909 Dr. Sluder wrote an article for *The New York State Journal of Medicine*, describing the anatomy and the clinical aspects of the sphenopalatine ganglion. He followed this a year later with an article in *The American Journal of Medical Science*, describing the pain of a headache in the lower half of the head, which he called "the syndrome of sphenopalatine ganglion neuralgia." This became known as the "Sluder Syndrome" and physicians still occasionally refer to it by that name. The syndrome is characterized by a single shooting pain at the base of the nose, radiating into the head and down the neck, to the shoulder, and sometimes even to the fingertips. Sluder treated this syndrome by blocking the ganglion, using a solution of cocaine or some other anesthetic. He tried destroying the ganglion with silver nitrate solution, but discovered the treatment had undesirable side effects, and recommended against it. Dr. Sluder is the father of the sphenopalatine ganglion blockade.

In the early 1920's Dr. Simon Ruskin, Dr. Milton Reder's brother-in-law, became interested in the sphenopalatine ganglion blockade. Dr. Ruskin was already a mature medical investigator who later became well-known for his development of two pharmaceuticals: calcium ascorbate and procaine penicillin. His interest in the blockade led him to the discovery that not only did it relieve head and facial pain, but it also worked for pain in the lumbosacral region. In 1925, in an article in *Laryngoscope* he wrote, "It is almost unbelievable that the pain of sciatica which has resisted every form of therapy, should yield within a few minutes to a local application of cocaine in the nose."

After Dr. Ruskin's writings and reports, others began to experiment with the procedure. Almost all reports were favorable. In 1930 Drs. H. Byrd and W. Byrd reported in the *Archives of Internal Medicine* that they gave 10,000 treatments to more than 2,000 patients and they reported relief of pain in approximately 75 percent of the cases.

In the early 1940s, Dr. J. Louis Amster suffered lumbo-sacral pain which he found could not be treated by ordinary methods. He heard of Dr. Ruskin, and went to him for treatment. His pain was relieved. Thereupon he began to use the procedure in his own practice.

In 1948, Amster presented a paper to the Anaesthesiology Section of the New York State Medical Society at its 142nd annual meeting. The paper was titled, "Sphenopalatine Ganglion Block for the Relief of Pain in Vascular and Muscular Spasm, with Special Reference to Lumbosacral Pain." He discussed 103 cases in which he used the SGB treatment and reported that lumbosacral pain was relieved in 90 percent of them.

It is interesting to note that Dr. Amster experimented with both pontocaine and cocaine for use in the treatment. Most of the doctors working in the field have concluded that cocaine is more effective, primarily because it works faster.

Dr. Amster concluded, "The results of topical application of an anaesthetic agent to the anterior or intra-nasal route are very striking, and with the simplicity of this method, combined with its safety, the spontaneous relief of pain (in many instances) and the absence of any toxic reactions, together with the economy of treatment, have earned the sphenopalatine block the name of an unbelievable therapeutic ganglion block."

In 1984 at the Fourth Annual World Congress of the International Association on the Study of Pain, Dr. R. S. Klein, of New York Medical School, gave a report which clearly and succinctly states the case for this form of therapy. The full report appears in Appendix III. It's worth reading.

On the basis of all this and other reports and studies, the Boston University School of Medicine and the Department of Medicine of Boston City Hospital undertook, in 1981, a scientific double-blind clinical test of the SGB for the treatment of acute low-back pain. This study is still in progress, but some interim results are available from the physicians in charge.

The protocol for the experiment involves ward patients 18 to 65 years of age who have come to the Boston City Hospital with complaints of low-back pain existing for one week or less, and who report that they were free of pain for at least a month prior to the acute episode. Patients are drawn from the Emergency Room, the Orthopedic Clinic, and the Medical Clinic. The nature of the treatment is explained in detail and they are invited to become subjects in the experiment. Those who consent are examined carefully in order to rule out causes which do not normally respond to the SGB.

All patients next complete a questionnaire in which they give their own subjective estimate of degree of pain and functional impairment. Thereafter they undergo a battery of physical tests for muscle spasm, sciatic irritation, range of spinal motion and ease of ambulation.

After completing the examination and the physical and written tests, 50 percent of the patients are given the SGB, using a 10 percent cocaine solution, and the other 50 percent are given the same procedure with water used as a placebo.

In the first group of fifteen patients, approximately 75 percent of those who received the cocaine SGB reported improvement, as against 25 percent who received the placebo. The overall test was approved for continuation.

As the experiment continues, the statistics seem to hold true. In early 1985 I received an unofficial report that approximately 75 percent of the patients treated with the standard SGB containing cocaine showed definite improvement in the relief of pain, as against 25 percent of the placebo group reporting similar results.

In some aspects the reports were even more remarkable

for the same period. For example, after a series of treatments the two groups were individually asked to make certain reports. Those treated with cocaine reported an improvement of more than 50 percent in the relief of their pain. The placebo group who experienced any relief reported only an 8 percent improvement.

Dr. J. C. Yang and others at the College of Physicians and Surgeons of Columbia University conducted an interesting experiment in the use of the SGB by actually creating pain and then treating it by the application of a 30 mg. solution of cocaine to the sphenopalatine ganglion. In this experiment they used healthy volunteers who agreed to test the procedure by allowing pain to be induced by the application of a tourniquet.

The tourniquet stops the blood flow and creates what is known as ischemic pain. It is the kind of pain that is found in certain diseases such as Raynaud's Disease. It is also found in frostbite and in angina pectoris.

Yang and his associates used a sixteen-patient double-blind test. They compared placebos against cocaine and they found a significant reduction in the pain when they used cocaine SGB.

CHAPTER III

Where the Miracles Take Place

The "house of miracles" occupies a portion of the first floor of 555 Park Avenue in Manhattan. From the time he first began to practice medicine as a specialist in ear, nose and throat problems, Dr. Reder has maintained offices on Park Avenue, although in three different locations. He closed his first Park Avenue office in 1941 when he went off to war. After the war ended, he opened his office in a new location, still on Park Avenue, but had to vacate it when the building was closed for extensive rehabilitation. For the past twenty years he has practiced at 555.

The office entrance is on Park Avenue and, to the consternation of many of his new patients arriving bent over with pain, two steps must be negotiated from the pavement to the entrance into the building. Patients suffering from sciatic pain, or foot and leg pains, struggle up these two steps, open the door, and then are confronted by five additional steep steps. To many who have barely managed to propel themselves to the location itself, this is truly the final challenge.

Many of Reder's patients have protested, "When I saw those five steps, I was ready to give up. I knew I could never make it." However, somehow the need to complete the pilgrimage provides the extra stamina to do just that.

A row of bells to one side of the doorway lists the names of several physicians who also occupy space on the first floor, although they are rarely in evidence and one sees only an occasional patient who is not Reder-bound. The bulk of the area is devoted to the chronic-pain practice of Dr. Milton Reder. To gain entrance to the offices, the visitor must ring the appropriate bell. A receptionist glances at the closed-circuit video monitor, and then presses a release button.

Once inside the entranceway, a right turn leads to an open area where a receptionist greets you. In fact, two receptionists spell each other. Sometimes their tours of duty overlap, so that at a given time both may be in evidence. Both are devoted to the doctor and carefully screen out curiosity seekers, exposé writers, and garden variety nuts.

Beyond the receptionists' desks (each has her own, even though they usually aren't present at the same time) is Dr. Reder's rather small treatment room where he performs the SGB procedure. That tiny office is furnished with oddly assorted chairs. One looks like an antique dental chair, another looks like a barber chair.

Dr. Reder sits in a swivel chair in front of his desk, with chairs flanking him on both sides. He can perform the procedure from either side, and frequently does, merely swiveling his chair from one side to the other.

As I noted before, no appointment is necessary. Dr. Reder arrives in his office very early in the morning. He insists he must accommodate those of his patients who travel considerable distances and would be unable to park their cars if they arrived after 8:00 a.m. Experienced patients—those who have been there at least once before—bypass the receptionist's desk and head directly for the inner sanctum. If the treatment chairs are unoccupied, they merely seat themselves and await the doctor's pleasure.

Once the applicators are in place, the patient is free to roam about the suite, sit, read, talk, or lie down. The large lounge, just off the doctor's treatment room, is furnished with an odd assortment of antique tables, chairs and couches which lend themselves to socializing while the patients wait to have the applicators removed. This is usually done after half an hour. Experience has convinced some patients that the results are improved if the applicators are retained for three quarters of an hour to an hour.

Because people arrive at a rate of approximately one every three minutes, at any given moment many patients are roaming about the suite, giving the offices somewhat the look of a party, albeit a somewhat eccentric one. A person entering the office for the first time, and wandering into the lounge, is startled to see as many as two dozen individuals in various relaxed postures, or standing, chatting in small groups, but all with what appear to be small knob-tipped wires emerging from their nostrils. Even more startling in this first impression is that no one seems to be aware of anything unusual. The newcomer quickly becomes accustomed to the sight and no longer sees it as extraordinary.

The large lounge is furnished in a most unconventional decor. The walls are covered with oil paintings, most of which are reproductions of familiar works of art currently hanging in museums. Tables of various sizes are covered with magazines, ranging from *Time* and *Newsweek* to medical journals.

Also on the tables are several sculpted busts of Dr.

Milton Reder. Only one is of great significance. It was done by Jose de Creeft, who is well known for his statue of Alice in Wonderland which delights the children playing in New York's Central Park. De Creeft was one of Dr. Reder's patients and, in gratitude for the relief of his pain, sculpted the head. A careful study of the sculpture is highly rewarding because de Creeft captured the spirit and essence of Dr. Reder. The face has an enigmatic half-smile, and an expression in the eyes which somehow manages to convey Reder's great concern for the welfare of his patients.

The entire scene at 555 Park Avenue—the furnishings, the patients with applicators in their nostrils, the chair miscellany, the paintings, and all the rest of the trappings remind me of one of the classic paintings of Hieronymus Bosch.

CHAPTER IV

Is the Cocaine Used in the Blockade Addictive?

From time to time accusations are leveled against the SGB that the cocaine used in the treatment disposes the patient to becoming an addict. For example, in a derogatory article in the May 14, 1984, issue of *New York* magazine, the writers quoted Dr. Mark Gold, head of the National Cocaine Help Line, as saying that "Dr. Reder's dosage would produce euphoria and dependence if used repeatedly."

This was a matter of some concern to me when I first heard of SGB, so I researched the subject. I concluded that Dr. Gold's statement is based on an erroneous conception of what the treatment really is.

All Those People

I interviewed literally hundreds of Dr. Reder's patients and I did not encounter one instance of anyone showing evidence of cocaine dependence, or who believed addiction had occurred.

Is the Cocaine Used in the Blockade Addictive?

Let's begin with my own personal experience. Over a period of several weeks I commuted to New York every Wednesday from my home in Philadelphia and remained until Sunday. During that time I took two treatments a day. This added up to ten treatments each week, spread over several weeks. I never sensed even the slightest hint of an addiction, although I observed myself very carefully for just that possibility.

For example, while I had no objection to the treatment, I also did not especially look forward to it, nor did I want to spend additional days in New York to take more of them.

Some patients I interviewed were in a pain crisis, and had been visiting Dr. Reder daily seven days a week for as long as ten to twelve weeks. One man had been coming five times a week for six months. No one ever showed any signs of addiction.

On the contrary, a number of patients told me, "I once went to Dr. Reder for almost a year before I got full relief from my condition. When I felt completely better, I stopped the treatments and I had no desire to return for more. In fact, I found it a relief not to have to make the long trip to Park Avenue any more. Furthermore, from my own knowledge I can say I experienced no symptoms of addiction at all."

To some degree or other, every long-term patient I interviewed said the same thing. The reason people use cocaine is to reach the euphoric state it offers. For example, *Merck's Manual* (the abbreviated desk reference book used by many physicians) has a section entitled, "Dependence of the Cocaine Type" (p. 1427) which summarizes cocaine addiction as follows:

> Cocaine is the prototype of a stimulant drug that in high doses produces euphoric excitement and, occasionally, halucinatory experiences. These properties are highly es-

> teemed by experienced drug users and lead to some degree of psychic dependence. Cocaine is probably the best example of a drug to which neither tolerance nor physical dependence develops, but to which psychic dependence develops that can lead to addiction.

There is absolutely no sense of euphoria from a Reder-administered sphenopalatine ganglion blockade. This conclusion is drawn not just from personal experience, but also from the time I have spent in Dr. Reder's office during the preparation of this book, observing hundreds of his patients. Most of them, after the treatment, present a rather listless appearance. They sit, recline, talk quietly, or just do nothing.

The National Institute on Drug Abuse (a federal agency) published an excellent monograph entitled "Cocaine, 1977." (If you want to obtain a copy, it is listed as "Research Monograph No. 13.") It is one of the most thorough studies on cocaine which I have examined during my intensive research on the subject. This book points out that people who use cocaine become talkative, energetic, and euphoric. My observation of Dr. Reder's patients revealed very few talkative ones; I saw no evidence of any of them becoming either unusually energetic or euphoric, symptoms of cocaine addiction.

The Placement of the Cocaine

Studies of cocaine users indicate that a very high percentage will, as they say, "snort" the drug. The procedure is to make a narrow line of powdered cocaine on a glass or mirrored surface, and then, using one of several methods, such as a rolled-up dollar bill, to inhale the line of cocaine through the tube into the nostrils.

The purpose of this procedure is to enable the cocaine to

coat the mucous membranes lining the nasal passages. This permits a quick entry into the blood stream. Some "coke" users will inject cocaine directly into a vein, but this method is comparatively rare. Customarily, the first method described here is the one most used.

The sphenopalatine ganglion blockade treatment carefully avoids contact between the cocaine-impregnated cotton and the mucous membranes, except for that small area of the membrane covering the sphenopalatine ganglion. No one has presented any evidence that the cocaine deposited on the ganglion is absorbed into the bloodstream.

If the treatment were designed to create euphoria, the treating physician would cause the saturated cotton pledget to contact the inner nasal membranes. This would give the full effect of cocaine absorption. As the true purpose of the treatment is to anesthetize the ganglion, and thus to relieve pain, the SGB physician avoids that contact.

The Difference in Dosage

Probably the major reason why it is erroneous to think that the SGB treatment depends upon the euphoric value of cocaine is because of the difference in dosages.

The addicted cocaine user puts about 50 mg. of cocaine into the "line" he inhales. Much, of course, depends upon the purity of the substance the user has obtained. In general, it is safe to say that the average user inhales about 25 mg. of pure cocaine each time. *Dr. Reder uses less than 5 mg. for all four applicators,* and not all of this is absorbed; a certain percentage remains on the cotton pledgets. It becomes obvious that the dosage is much less than 10 percent of the amount an habitual cocaine user inhales to achieve a "high."

This is a good place to explain exactly how Dr. Reder makes use of the cocaine. First, he obtains a small bottle of cocaine in a water solution. He uses four cotton-wrapped applicators for each treatment. He takes one applicator, dips it into the bottle of cocaine solution, then takes the other three applicators and squeezes all four together to moisten them from the contents of the single saturated one. This type of applicator preparation considerably reduces the overall dosage. When the four applicators ultimately come into contact with the ganglion, each one holds only one-fourth of the original dosage, but this is enough to produce anesthetization of the ganglion.

Applied in this way, not all of the solution is passed on to the body. In fact, most physicians who know anything about the treatment believe that only a small portion of the original dosage of cocaine is available, the remainder being absorbed by the cotton itself.

For those of my readers who are unfamiliar with just what quantity a milligram represents, let me illustrate: It is one-thousandth of one-thirtieth of an ounce! So the somewhat less than 5 mg. total that is used in the sphenopalatine ganglion blockade is truly infinitesimal, far too small to create addiction, and much too weak to achieve a "high."

The Cost Factor

I think it is interesting to make a comparison between the cost to the patient of the Reder treatment and the cost of cocaine to a habitual cocaine user. Dr. Reder charges $25 per treatment (not per applicator). Cocaine on the street with an average purity of 50 percent will run $250 per gram. A gram produces about twenty "lines" for the coke-sniffer. The average user will sniff three times per evening per nostril, a total of six "lines." This brings the cost per user per night to about $75 for an evening's high.

If the amount of cocaine used in the SGB approximated the quantity used by the cocaine addict, obviously the charge per treatment would have to be considerably higher. This type of evidence may be more economic than scientific, but it certainly has its place in an evaluation of the dangers of addiction merely from the SGB itself.

Finally, here's the bottom line: It costs Dr. Reder $35 per bottle of the solution he uses. He gets 140 applications out of each bottle, which comes to twenty-five cents per treatment. The idea that twenty-five cents worth of cocaine could have an addictive effect is preposterous.

The Yang-Columbia University Study

Dr. J. C. Yang is an assistant professor of Anesthesiology at Columbia University Medical School. Dr. W. C. Clark is a Research Scientist at the New York State Psychiatric Institute. In 1982 Yang and Clark, together with some assistants, decided to test the pain-relieving effects of intra-nasal cocaine to determine how much of the relief was produced by the euphoric effect cocaine users experience.

The experiment is described in *Anesthesia and Analgesia*, the journal of the International Anesthesia Research Society. The specific article is entitled "Effect of Intranasal Cocaine on Experimental Pain in Man." (see Volume 61 at page 358.)

Yang and Clark used sixteen male volunteers who were told that they would be treated intra-nasally with either cocaine or a saline solution. The subjects were not told which solution would be used at any given time. To test the relative pain-killing effects of cocaine and the placebo, ischemic pain was induced in the subject. This type of pain is produced by obstructing the flow of arterial blood, a condition which results naturally from frostbite and from angina pectoris. In the laboratory, ischemic pain is produced by placing a tight tourniquet around the upper arm.

The subjects were required to fill out a series of pain

questionnaires, including the Speilburger State Anxiety Inventory Test, and the Clark Drug Reaction Checklist.

The subjects of the experiment had to decide if the pain was lessened by the introduction of the solution into the nose, and also had to describe how the pain was reduced or eliminated. Yang and Clark reached two conclusions.

First, evaluation of the subjects' responses indicated the pain was reduced when cocaine was used, in contrast to the effect of the saline solution.

Perhaps more importantly, they concluded, "It is unlikely euphoria made any important contribution to the analgesic effect because the psychological changes were minimal. . . ."

The work of Yang and Clark confirmed that the sphenopalatine ganglion blockade does not relieve pain by creating a euphoric condition in the body. It works because cocaine anesthetizes the ganglion and thus blocks the pain.

Blood Pressure Peculiarity

Finally, in my research into the possibility that the Reder treatment worked because of cocaine-induced euphoria, I encountered the following phenomenon: A moderate amount of cocaine taken through the snorting method will definitely *raise* the blood pressure of the user. (See the discussion on page 10 of the monograph "Cocaine, 1977" from the National Institute On Drug Abuse.) However, there is evidence showing that the Reder treatment in fact *lowers* the blood pressure. Some of Dr. Reder's patients come to him specifically to maintain a healthy blood pressure without having to use other medications.

It is clear that a world of difference exists between the cocaine treatment used in the sphenopalatine ganglion blockade and the addict's snorting of cocaine to achieve a "high."

CHAPTER V

A Day in the Life of the Miracle Worker

Dr. Reder awakens sometime between 3:00 a.m. and 4:00 a.m. Like many older people, he has difficulty sleeping long stretches at a time. However, during the day he is likely to doze off at his desk if there are no patients waiting for him. Additionally, he takes a nap during the lunch break. But it's early to rise for the Reders. This particular morning, a run-of-the-mill day, a severe pain in the heel of his foot wakes him. He knows it is probably caused by his diabetes, but it may also be related to the fact that he suffers from a spinal stenosis (a narrowing of the spine, impinging on the sciatic nerve).

He takes two Tylenol tablets to relieve the pain in his foot. Normally, he would give himself an SGB treatment, but he doesn't keep the medication at home. If he anticipates a problem, he brings some home with him the night before.

After the Tylenol takes effect, he feels a little better and sits down for the breakfast his wife always gets up early enough to prepare for him. He has a sliced orange, an egg, toast and "coffee." For a variety of reasons, he avoids caffeine, and always drinks Sanka.

His friend, Dr. Theodore Ehrenreich, picks him up at about 6:00 a.m. Ehrenreich is a well-known pathologist in the city of New York, and at one time was on the staff of Office of the Medical Examiner. Now in private practice, he specializes in forensic pathology, especially matters dealing with certain types of chemically caused disabling occupational diseases.

Dr. Ehrenreich is a Reder patient. He has suffered with chronic back pain for many years. Many mornings when he drops Dr. Reder off, he takes a treatment before going to his own office.

If Dr. Ehrenreich does not come by, Dr. Reder will take a taxi. In any event, he tries to arrive at his office by 6:30 a.m. Many of his patients drive in from New Jersey and Connecticut, and other distant places, and the cost of parking in the area is at least $12.50. Dr. Reder likes to save his patients that $12.50. Before eight o'clock they can legally park their cars on Park Avenue in front of his office.

When he arrives, usually at least one or two patients are already waiting for him in front of his office. These people are long-termers. They have all been there before, and Dr. Reder can rapidly insert the applicators so that they can begin their half-hour treatment, after which they will return to the inner room to have them removed.

In the early morning, there is an occasional lull between patients, and Reder will glance through *The New York Times* while he waits. This morning, having arisen especially early, he nods off for a five-minute catnap. Now patients begin to arrive again.

By 9:30 a.m. the patient traffic is heavy. The doctor knows all of his patients and remembers their ailments—no small accomplishment, considering the vast scope of his practice. He asks one, "And how is the pain down the leg?"

The patient replies, "What pain? I haven't felt a pain since you started the treatments."

Another patient enters. Dr. Reder asks, "Are the headaches lightening up?"

He nods approvingly at the reply, "They are much better—not all gone, but I can live with them. As long as I come to you, I feel like a human being."

About 10:30 a.m. the Back Stage Deli, located on Lexington Avenue near 62nd Street, sends over a standing order in a cardboard carton of Sanka and a bun. Dr. Reder will sip some of the Sanka and nibble at the bun over the next hour.

A steady stream of patients passes through the office. Every once in a while one of them has something unusual to tell, and Reder draws them out for my benefit, so I can record the story. Here's a woman who has come in because of lower back pain. He greets her jovially, saying, "This man is checking on me. Tell him about the first time you came."

The woman, a middle-aged patrician, tells me, "A few years ago I came here because I was at my wits' end. I have myasthenia gravis. One of the results of this disease is that my eyelids close. When I arrived, my eyes were almost completely closed. I couldn't keep the eyelids open at all. My sister had to bring me in.

"I told Dr. Reder that I had come to him as a last resort. He said, 'I don't know what this will do for you. But let's give it a try.' Then he gave me the standard treatment. I was the most surprised person in the world when, after having the applicators in my nose for only about fifteen minutes, my lids started to lift. Before I knew it, I had normal vision and my eyelids were working as well as anyone else's."

I wanted to know why she was there now and she explained, "I occasionally have lower back pain, and I come for that."

I asked, "Did your eyelids have lasting effect from the treatments?"

She answered, "The treatment is good for a month or two, and then I have to come back. But it's wonderful just to know that if it gets really bad, I can come here for relief. One doctor suggested I should have them sewed open so that they will stay up, but I couldn't stand the thought of having a needle go through my eyelids. The doctor told me it wouldn't be painful, but just thinking about having my eyes always open made me shudder. I would rather see Dr. Reder when necessary. He's done wonders for me."

Her applicators are now inserted, and she is off to the lounge, to wait out her thirty minutes in the company of other patients. A new patient takes her place.

By 12:30 p.m. the patient traffic gradually slows down. People who are familiar with the doctor's routine know that he stops treating patients at 12:30 p.m., because he closes the office at one o'clock and doesn't re-open until three o'clock.

Around 12:30 p.m. the Back Stage Deli delivers a carton of Sanka and a "scoop bagel." This is the standard bagel with much of the center scooped out. Dr. Reder believes the center isn't good for him. The bagel has been filled with cream cheese and lox and he eats one-half of it that day, and puts the remainder in a small Sanyo refrigerator in his inner office. He will eat the second half the next day. Yul Brynner had the refrigerator installed because he wanted a place to keep his Gatorade cold when he visited the doctor for treatment, and he also wanted to give Reder a gift.

Sometime after one o'clock, when all the morning patients have gone and he has finished his half of a scoop bagel and Sanka, Reder goes into the large lounge, where he takes a nap on one of the couches. He sleeps as long as he can, but usually not more than an hour.

Office hours resume at three o'clock. By this time a number of people have congregated in the outer waiting room, impatiently waiting their turn for pain-relief therapy. Sometimes Dr. Reder makes himself available by 2:45 p.m., because it bothers him to ignore suffering people, or to keep them waiting unnecessarily.

Today is a special day because Dr. Milton A. Reder will arrive at four o'clock. Dr. Reder's handsome, thirty-two-year-old son stands six-feet four-inches tall, and the father's pride in him is immediately evident. The senior Reder will tell you how his son was admitted to a very special school for gifted children when he was three years old. Young Reder attended Johns Hopkins undergraduate and then Johns Hopkins Medical School. Upon graduation, he accepted an internship, and then a residency, at Boston Medical College. His initial specialty was in Internal Medicine and he is certified by the American Board of Internal Medicine.

He explains, "I spent many years watching people crawl in, limp in, or be carried into my father's office. I observed the treatment, and watched them walk out on their own. I was deeply impressed by what I saw and made it a point to learn to administer the treatment so I could use it when it appeared appropriate."

Young Dr. Reder, in his early days of practice, developed an interest in the treatment of arthritis. It was only natural for him to test the sphenopalatine ganglion blockade to discover if it would have any effect on arthritis. He found it to be an excellent treatment. When he opened his office at 28 Manchester Road, Brookline, Massachusetts, he offered the SGB treatment to his patients for relief for all types of pain, and he continues to do so.

He comes to New York once or twice a week to help his father with the patient load. When patient traffic reaches a peak in the afternoon, the son helps his father with the insertions. He also wraps the cotton around the applicator tips, helps sterilize instruments, and generally makes himself useful in any way he can. A few of the long-time patients who have become accustomed to the elder Dr. Reder will not let the young man treat them, but this is rare. Most of the patients accept either doctor. Observing them both, I saw very little difference in skill or manner.

As I watch, a new patient enters and the older doctor questions her. Having satisfied himself that she qualifies for the treatment, he inserts the applicators. She complains, "I feel something bitter in my throat."

Dr. Reder says reassuringly, "That's natural. Some fluids are running down into your throat. Here, take this." He hands her a wrapped butterscotch candy and continues, "I keep these on my desk for patients like you. You'll get used to that feeling, and you won't have to have the candy after a while, but right now I want you to suck on it. It neutralizes the unpleasant taste in your throat."

The new patient asks, "What do you charge for the treatment, doctor?"

Reder replies, "The charge is $25 per treatment."

I asked him how long he had been charging $25 and he answered, "Ever since I started my practice."

I stared at him unbelievingly. "Haven't you heard of inflation?"

His eyes twinkled. "I think $25 is enough for the treatment. I don't need more. I don't want more."

I turned to the younger Reder and asked, "What do you charge?" He replied, "I charge $25. That seems to be the family tradition. I certainly don't want to mess with success."

Office traffic begins to slacken around 5:30 p.m. Patients

know that Dr. Reder likes to close up at six o'clock, so they must arrive before 5:30 p.m. in order to complete a treatment. He rarely actually leaves by six o'clock, because there are always a few patients who feel the need for another five minutes or so. He is a kindly man who empathizes with his patients' needs, so he hurries no one. But finally, the last patient has left and the doctor is ready to close up for the day. However, this is not the end for him.

In front of the building a limousine, sent by Daniel K. Ludwig, awaits Dr. Reder's departure. (Mr. Ludwig, a Reder patient, is one of the richest men in the world.) He requires several treatments during the week, but does not come to the office. Dr. Reder still makes house calls when he feels a patient requires it. He carries with him a supply of sterile applicators and the medical solution he needs. Mr. Ludwig is not Dr. Reder's only house call, but he is the one tonight.

When his visit is finished, the limousine will return the doctor to his home. He eats dinner, and then watches TV if any of his patients has informed him of an appearance on the tube.

He says, "I really don't care for television, but I don't like to disappoint a patient who has told me about a TV appearance. I try to make it a point to remember to watch at that time."

When I asked him if there was anyone in particular he watches for, he replied, "George C. Scott, George Burns, Phil Silvers, Alan King, Dom De Luise, Yul Brynner, Steve Lawrence and Edie Gorme, Rodney Dangerfield, David Susskind and David Brenner."

"Are all those people your patients?" I wanted to know.

"Well, all of them have been to see me at one time or another. Some more often than others, but all of them have been patients."

If he has nothing he wants to watch on TV, he is in bed shortly after 8:30 p.m. Otherwise, he retires after the show. Rarely does he go to bed later than ten o'clock. He has to be in the office by 6:30 a.m. and that makes for a long day!

CHAPTER VI

The Members of the Healing Arts Profession

Approximately 5 percent of Dr. Reder's patients are members of the healing arts professions. These include physicians, nurses, dentists, psychologists, and others. Some are general practitioners and some are well-known specialists. They are neurologists, rheumatologists, pediatricians, geriatricians, hematologists, and pathologists.

Basically, the pattern of trauma is much the same among the members of the profession as it is among laymen. Probably the only difference is that, instead of hearing, "I have this terrible pain in my lower back," Dr. Reder gets technical jargon and self-diagnosis.

As I speak to the professionals, in place of the common "I have this shooting pain down my right leg," or "I have this sharp pain in my back," I hear instead, "thoracic scoliosis, spinal stenosis, displaced annulis fibrosis." Where a layman says, "I felt an awful pain suddenly on the right side of my back," the professional will say, "I had a spasm of the erector spinae muscle." Or the pain may be described as "in the iliopsoas muscle." The physicians talk about "ankylosing spondylitis" or "spondylolisthesis."

Whatever they say, it all means the same. They have pain; they hurt; they've tried all the standard weapons in the arsenal of medicine and they still hurt. Now they're trying Dr. Reder, as a court of last resort.

In discussing the phenomenon of the sphenopalatine ganglion blockade with the professionals, a uniform comment becomes apparent. "I could fully understand how the anesthetization of the sphenopalatine ganglion would help to relieve pain, or even eliminate it, in the head or face. However, I cannot comprehend how the anesthetizing of that ganglion does anything for pain in the lower portion of the body. But I have to admit, it works!"

While gathering material for this book, I taped most of the conversations I had with Reder's patients. I interviewed a widely-known physician who is a specialist in an important branch of medicine, and on the staff of the major medical institutes in New York City. This physician has access to almost any specialist in the world. The following is a verbatim transcript of our interview:

Q. What condition brought you to Dr. Reder?

A. Chronic relapsing pericarditis.

Q. Would you please explain that condition to me?

A. It is an inflammation of the pericardium.

Q. And that is—?

A. The pericardium is the closed membranous sac enveloping the heart. The base is attached to the central tendon of the diaphragm and its apex surrounds the great vessels which arise from the base of the heart. It consists of an outer fibrous coat, and an inner serous coat. It is sometimes referred to by laymen as the envelope which holds the heart.

Q. And what are the symptoms of that condition?

A. Some fever, a severe precordial pain and tenderness, some coughing and a rapid pulse.

Q. But essentially your problem is pain?

A. Yes. That's it.

Q. When did this problem begin?

A. January, 1984.

Q. Was it diagnosed quickly?

A. Not really. It took six months before it was accurately diagnosed because I had no symptoms of illness—just the pain.

Q. Where was the pain? Can you describe it?

A. The pain was typical of pericarditis. It was, in fact, treated as such by the physicians who examined me. The picture of the condition was there, but the objective tests were negative. They didn't develop any positive signs on the electrocardiogram or the echo cardiogram until about six months after the pain started. It was a very atypical case.

Q. What treatment was administered initially?

A. I received all the standard treatments for it, and they all failed. I received all the non-steroidal, anti-inflammatory medications. I responded slightly to a course of pregnisone, which is a form of cortisone. Unfortunately, that response only lasted a short time. I relapsed again with severe chest pains.

Q. What did the doctors do then?

A. They upped the dose of pregnisone to as high as 50 mg. This still failed to bring me any relief. I was maintained on a chronic dosage of pregnisone of 40 mg. for several months. I got no relief, no benefit, but I got a lot of unhappy side effects from the pregnisone.

Q. How did you hear about Dr. Reder?

A. I had heard about him earlier from a physician friend who sent my wife to him. My friend actually came in and took one of the treatments. He reported to me that it was not uncomfortable and he suggested I ought to try it because everything else had failed.

Q. When did you take your first treatment?

A. Christmas Eve, 1984.

Q. Did you get any response after the first treatment?

A. I would say it changed the nature of the pain. Instead of the aching, grinding sensation in my chest, I had only a tingling sensation for several hours after the treatment. The actual pain was relieved for a few hours.

Q. What did you do then?

A. I began to come here every day. Sometimes I took two treatments in one day. I learned that if I came regularly, I didn't have any pain at all.

Q. Generally speaking, how do you feel now?

A. I feel human. I feel free of pain. What troubles me is that I know all too well that this treatment eliminates the pain, but it doesn't relieve the condition that causes it. Even so, getting rid of the pain does let me do my work and treat my patients.

Q. Do you understand how this treatment works relative to your own problem?

A. Frankly, no. I really don't understand how, or why, it works, but I'm just thankful that it does!

This interview was typical of the thinking of a professional with regard to the sphenopalatine ganglion block, Dr. Reder's unorthodox but many times successful treatments.

CHAPTER VII

In Which I Relate Some of the Miracles I Have Heard

Before discussing the specific cases that I regard as "miracles" I want to make it clear that not all of Dr. Reder's treatments result in miracles, or even near-miracles. The following is a typical story told me by one of Dr. Reder's patients:

"I had this pain down my right leg. I could hardly walk and it hurt me even when I was sitting or sleeping. The pain was intense. First I managed to control it by taking Tylenol or aspirin but after a while that stopped helping. I started taking stronger medicines prescribed by an assortment of doctors. Then they didn't help, either.

"I was in severe pain all the time. I couldn't work. I couldn't think. I couldn't read. I couldn't even concentrate on television. All I could think about was how much I hurt. My life, awake or asleep, revolved around pain. The only thing I wanted from life was to find a way to make it stop hurting.

"I tried everything. I went to orthopedic physicians, chiropractors, acupuncturists—you name it. If I heard about anybody who might be any good in the relief of sciatic pain, I ran there. I spoke about it to everybody I knew. Nobody helped!

"One day, one of the doctors I visited suggested, almost apologetically, that I visit Dr. Reder. I remember he told me, 'Milton Reder's treatment is unorthodox, but I happen to know that he sometimes can relieve pain where no other treatment helps. You should give it a try.'

"The doctor gave me Dr. Reder's phone number and I called to make an appointment. I would have gone to a witch doctor if I thought it might help. At the time I did not know that appointments were unnecessary. I showed up at Dr. Reder's office one day at three o'clock, and he took my full history. Then he gave me my first treatment, placing the applicators into my nose.

"The very first treatment gave me slight relief. I'm not even sure you could call it relief—maybe it was just psychological. Anyway, I felt a little less pain. It was hardly enough to warrant continuing the treatments, but I was desperate by now. I figured this was as good as anything else I had tried up to then.

"Dr. Reder suggested I take a course of treatments on a daily basis. I started coming here every day, taking two treatments each day. At first, I didn't really notice any relief from pain, but it seemed to me it was doing me some good. I was sleeping better at night, and I could even sit and watch television for five or ten minutes and forget the pain. At the end of about a month, I would say that Dr. Reder's treatments had made the pain bearable. He didn't make it go away.

"I would be lying if I told you I was pain-free. I'm still not without pain, and I've been coming off and on for two years. What's important is that Dr. Reder's treatment makes the pain bearable. The edge is blunted, and the pain is no longer so sharp that I can't think about anything else.

"I no longer think of suicide, although I have to tell you that many times I was on the edge of it, when I felt I just couldn't stand another second of pain. My life just didn't seem worth living. What Dr. Reder has accomplished is to make the quality of my life vastly better. Even though I still suffer pain, I can handle it—live with it—now. And when it gets too bad, at least I know I have some place to come for relief."

The foregoing represents a common story among Dr. Milton Reder's patients. The Reder treatment reduces pain to a reasonable, bearable state. On the other hand, in some cases, Dr. Reder's treatment, whether it be for pain or for some other problem, actually improves the condition to such an extent and with such speed that the word "miracle" seems to apply. The following are some of the stories of "miracles" which I collected from my interviews:

The Case of the Lost Voice

Ruth Rosen is an attractive young woman, thin and well built. She is twenty years old and had led a normal life, free of physical problems. She worked as a secretary and her hobby was singing in her congregation choir. One day she lost her voice.

The doctors diagnosed it as "spastic dysphonia."

The doctors always have scientific names for everything, but that doesn't necessarily mean they know what the problem really is, or what to do about it. For example, "spastic" simply means that something results from a spasm. In short, it wasn't caused by a bruise, a cut, or even aging. It was created by a spasm. "Dysphonia" means that the voice (phonia) has been impaired or disabled or become morbid. In short, it means something went wrong with the voice.

Ruth has no idea of any possible event which could have caused her to lose her voice. She had no accident, no trauma, no blow, no psychological shock, nothing which could have produced the loss of her voice. She simply opened her mouth to say something, and found she had no voice.

She began a round of visits to doctors. Her general practitioner recommended an ear, nose and throat specialist. The latter, finding nothing wrong, sent her to a neurologist. The neurologist, still unable to find a causative factor, sent her to a psychiatrist.

She claims to have visited half the medical practitioners in New York City. No one could help her. Somewhere along the line, someone suggested a neurosurgeon might be able to help, but the most optimistic estimate of success for this type of surgery was about 10 percent. She didn't like the odds.

Finally, she heard about Dr. Milton Reder. In desperation, she came at last to 555 Park Avenue and viewed with astonishment the assortment of characters with applicators sticking out of their noses. She felt she had wandered into some surrealistic movie set. She nervously went in to see the doctor.

Dr. Reder listened attentively while the friend who accompanied her explained the problem, and told of her medical history. He looked dubious but at last he made his usual comment: "Let's give it a try. It can't hurt you. Since your problem lies near the sphenopalatine ganglion, we might get some result. The spasm which causes your loss of voice may be stopped by the blockade, and you'll be home free."

Gently Dr. Reder inserted the applicators into her nostrils. She sat nervously waiting, with no real hope. She felt sure that once again she was wasting her time. The best voice doctors in metropolitan New York had checked her carefully and been unable to help. How could this old man, who could hardly even rise to his feet, help her when everyone else had failed?

When she started to get up from her chair, Dr. Reder told her to sit quietly. He observed her carefully. Then, to her great surprise, he urged, "Let's give it a try. Talk to me."

Feeling certain it was a waste of time and effort, she opened her mouth and said, "I don't think . . ." An expression of intense surprise crossed her face. Her voice box was operational! She could hear her own voice! She could speak. Other patients who had been listening to her story with great interest began to applaud. Everyone there was encouraging her. They urged, "Keep talking! Don't stop. Dr. Reder has performed another miracle!"

And talk she did. Her voice was hoarse and much lower in pitch than it had been before she lost it, but it was a voice. She could speak. Her delight defies description. She felt like she was floating on Cloud Nine.

At Dr. Reder's suggestion—to avoid any loss of momentum—she began to come every day for treatment. At the end of the first week, after seven treatments, her voice was almost normal.

Not wanting to take any chances of relapse, she continued with Dr. Reder, coming two or three times each week for several weeks. As she says, "I not only got my old voice back, but it had a greater range than it ever had before. After Dr. Reder's treatments, I began to hit notes that I could never have reached before. I have no doubt but that these treatments have improved my singing voice."

What is Dr. Reder's explanation? He says, "The spheno-palatine ganglion controls a lot of muscles, many of which we don't really comprehend. The anesthetizing of the ganglion allows the muscles that are controlled by it to relax completely. A more relaxed muscle will function better than a muscle that is tight or rigid."

Many physicians will disagree with that explanation, and will disbelieve the entire occurrence, but the young woman who recovered her voice is a believer! She doesn't care what anyone else thinks. She knows a miracle when she has one!

The Pain Comes Later

Ray Thomas is a handsome forty-year-old man with a thick head of hair. Women find him attractive. However, he avoids women as much as he avoids other types of involvement, because he suffers from carotid sinus syndrome. I asked him to describe his condition for me.

"There is a carotid artery on each side of the neck. The carotid artery splits as it goes toward the brain. At one point a small organ regulates the blood pressure and the pulse rate. If anything traumatizes that regulator point, the blood presure can drop sharply, causing blackouts. This happened to me one day while I was shaving. I was standing there shaving, feeling in perfectly good health, when all of a sudden I blacked out and dropped to the floor, hitting my chin on the washstand as I fell. My jaw ached for two weeks afterward."

I asked, "Does this condition cause pain?"

"No," he replied wryly, "it only hurts afterwards, if you faint and hit something."

Ray Thomas promptly saw his physician. The doctor recommended a cardiologist. After a complete examination, the cardiologist suggested he try to avoid touching his neck because pressure on the carotid artery is a causative factor in the syndrome. Thereafter, he carefully avoided applying any pressure to his neck. One day, while in the barber's chair being shaved, the barber touched the area around the carotid artery, and again Mr. Thomas blacked out. The blackout lasted a substantial period of time and the frightened barber called the paramedics. Ray Thomas woke up in the hospital.

From that time on, he was super careful. He didn't touch his neck, and he tried very hard to prevent anyone else from touching his neck. Then it happened! Ray said, "I was sitting in my chair reading. I'm sure I didn't touch my neck at all. No one was even close to me. Suddenly I blacked out."

Thomas went to see the cardiologist again. The doctor suggested the possibility of surgical intervention. Ray Thomas felt negative about this approach. He felt such surgery too dangerous to attempt except as a last resort. In addition, the cardiologist would give him no real assurance that it would help. It was just another possible way to go. After considering the operation, he rejected it.

Someone suggested he see Dr. Milton Reder. At his first visit, Dr. Reder explained that it was possible the sphenopalatine ganglion blockade would eliminate the carotid sinus syndrome. Reder said he had encountered a few similar cases where the blockade worked, but he could give him no guarantees. Thomas observed the patients walking around with applicators in their noses, spoke to some of them and, reassured by their stories, decided to try it himself. To his great relief, the treatments worked.

He told me, "I never had another episode after I began coming to Dr. Reder. At first, I came every day. Then I dropped back to once a week. Now I come once a month, and believe me, I wouldn't consider missing that treatment. I'm not even careful about my neck now, and I still haven't had a recurrence.

"In fact, I even experimented a little. I squeezed my neck in different places, and nothing happened. I really believe that these treatments have cured me."

The Man Who Returned from Tokyo

George Gunther is in his early sixties, and he suffers from cluster headaches. George told me, "I used to get these headaches in batches. Suddenly one Monday morning I'd get a headache and I would be in severe pain all day. It might come back on Tuesday or Wednesday, and again on Friday. Then it would stop. In other words, it came in clusters."

As I had discovered in other interviews, most of Dr. Reder's patients were quite knowledgeable about the possible causes of their pain. In this instance, George favored me with a lecture on the subject of cluster headaches.

The pain of a cluster headache centers around one of the eyes. The pupil contracts, the eye becomes red and weepy, and the eyelid droops. Vision blurs.

The cluster headache is usually accompanied by severe and intense pain. Most sufferers of headaches want to lie down quietly, but the victim of cluster headache needs to be physically active, and may, in extreme cases, be driven to pound on walls, or throw things.

The true cluster headache is relatively rare, occurring in less than one percent of the population, and attacking men more than women. It has also been called Horton's Syndrome, migrainous neuralgia, and histamine cephalgia.

George told me, "The headaches come in clusters. Sometimes I get one over a period of a month or two, and then I might go several months without an attack. I learned to dread certain times of the day, because those were the time when an attack was likely to begin. Often I would have an attack about an hour and a half after I fell asleep. If I was in the middle of a cluster, I'd be afraid to take a nap during the day, because that was when the pain would strike."

No one seems to know the causes of cluster headaches. Histamines and alcohol can trigger one. And treatment is very difficult. Migraine is usually stress-induced, but cluster strikes even a completely relaxed person. Therefore, it doesn't respond to such therapies as biofeedback or psychotherapy.

At first he took pain killers—aspirin, Tylenol, percadan, and the rest of the spectrum of analgesics. These helped in the beginning. "Gradually," he continued, "I started to feel the pain no matter what I took. Nothing helped any more. Nothing worked. I tried taking larger doses, but it didn't help. Sometimes I took a large enough dose to put me to sleep, but the pain hung on."

George started the customary trek from doctor to doctor and from pain clinic to pain clinic. He tried biofeedback, hypnosis, and all the cures and any palliatives that anyone mentioned to him. No matter what he tried, the headaches got stronger and stronger, driving him to desperation. They came with increasing frequency, and all his controls were weakening. At his wit's end, he finally visited Dr. Reder.

This was one of the few cases I encountered where Dr. Reder said, "I believe my treatment will take care of your problem. It is very good for headaches. In fact, that is one of the most responsive conditions."

Usually Dr. Reder is very guarded in his prognosis. I have never heard him tell a patient positively that the treatment would help; usually he says, "Let's give it a try."

George Gunther began his course of treatments with Dr. Reder. "To my enormous relief, it worked like magic. I came there an utterly desperate man. I was in the middle of a cluster headache. I had had one all day, and I had tried everything I could think of.

"It was late in the afternoon when I walked into Dr. Reder's office, and by then my pain was so agonizing I could hardly think straight. I told the doctor my full story, and then he placed the applicators into my nose.

"I don't think it took more than ten minutes before I was certain my pain was growing less. I felt like I had had a vise around my head, and then someone began to release the tension on it. By the end of the first treatment, I felt like a human being again."

George Gunther now visits Dr. Reder three times a week. He has no headaches if he sticks to this regimen. However, his business requires him to travel frequently, and sometimes he has to be away for a few weeks. During these periods of absence from New York, if he feels the slightest twinge of a beginning cluster headache, he leaves wherever he is to fly to New York and Dr. Reder.

One day he found himself in Tokyo at a business luncheon with some Japanese, where he was in the midst of closing a deal to import electronic components. Halfway through the meal, he felt a twinge in his head.

George Gunther reports, "I knew I could stand the headache that was coming, for the rest of the day, and maybe even for the next day, until I got back to the United States. However, I was terrified that somehow, once I allowed the strength of the headache to increase, it might be stronger than Dr. Reder's medicine could relieve. I couldn't face the possibility I might go back to the way I had been before Reder. I had an overwhelming urge to return to the U.S.A. for a treatment as quickly as possible. Dr. Reder's medicine had to stay in control of the headaches. I don't know if that makes any sense to you, but that's the way I felt."

In short, George Gunther rose from his seat in the restaurant, excused himself, returned to his hotel, and called the airline for the earliest departure. Within half an hour, he was in a taxi bound for the airport. There he boarded a flight to the United States. His 747 landed at Kennedy the next morning, and he took a cab directly to Dr. Reder's office.

He says, "I reached 555 Park Avenue at about eight o'clock in the morning. I could hardly wait to rush in, and the most glorious sight I ever saw in my life was Dr. Reder sitting in his chair in front of his desk preparing applicators for use. I could hardly wait to get the treatment. My headache hadn't hit me hard yet, but I could tell it was on the way. I could feel the slight tightening sensation in my scalp which always heralded the imminent arrival of pain. I think my anticipation of reaching Dr. Reder had kept it at bay on my way from Tokyo. In any event, within minutes after my arrival in Reder's office, I was seated in the chair and the applicators had been inserted. The headache never arrived, and I haven't had one since then."

CHAPTER VIII

More Case Histories for Skeptics

The Woman Who Wanted to Kill Herself

I studied the woman before me. She was in her late fifties or early sixties. Her gray hair was worn coiled regally on top of her head like a crown. Her glance was sharp, and her manner brusque. When I questioned her about the nature of the problem that brought her to Dr. Reder, she answered shortly, "Tic douloureux."

I asked her for a definition.

She snapped at me, "Mr. Gerber, I'm no doctor. Ask Dr. Reder."

I did, and he explained to me that it was a paroxysmal neuralgia of the trigeminal nerve. In short, it was a kind of spasm or convulsion of the trigeminal nerve itself, which caused severe pain in the head.

The woman had suffered from tic douloureux for twenty years, during which time she had tried everything. When I induced her to discuss her problem with me, she told me that she had seriously considered suicide because she just couldn't go on living with the sudden convulsive and excruciatingly painful seizures that ripped through her head. The doctors had no difficulty diagnosing the condition, but could offer no help.

Approximately five years ago she had heard of Dr. Reder's treatment and, as a last resort, snatched at the faint hope of relief and journeyed to 555 Park Avenue. I asked her how it had worked for her.

She replied, "It happened that I came to him during a period of remission. At that moment I was not having a seizure, so I wasn't in much pain. He gave me a treatment and I had no pain for a day or two. I came back for another treatment. Again I had no convulsion, so I didn't have pain.

"I began to take some real interest in Dr. Reder's procedure, for the first time. I decided to test how long it would keep me from a seizure. I began to visit him every other day. For the first time in my life I passed several weeks without a seizure or pain. Then I had some business on the West Coast, and I didn't see Dr. Reder for about two weeks. Sure enough, at the end of the second week I had another seizure. It wasn't one of the worst I've ever had, but it wasn't good either. I came back to Dr. Reder, and since then I never go a week without a treatment."

Half in jest, half seriously, I asked, "Dr. Reder's getting old. What will you do when he retires?"

She smiled for the first time in our interview, and replied, "I'm way ahead of you on that one. Don't think I didn't think about it. I have a list of all the doctors who give the treatment, and if Dr. Reder closes up shop, I'll go to one of the others. Thank God, he has trained other doctors in the procedure."

The Man Who Couldn't Stop Hiccuping

Seth Samuels is a structural engineer who tests metals, sometimes in the laboratory and sometimes on a structure itself. One day he had an attack of hiccups. He had had them before and had developed a couple of remedies that usually worked for him. He drank a glass of water slowly, sipping and trying not to breathe. It didn't work. He took a plastic bag and breathed into it until he filled the bag with carbon dioxide.

He told me, "In the past, using the bag almost always worked like a charm. I have been subject to attacks of hiccuping for a long time, and over the years I learned how to deal with it. This time, for some reason, nothing worked."

The hiccups continued for twenty-four hours, and finally Seth went to a doctor, who gave him a prescription for something. What it was, he doesn't know. He had it filled, tried it, and kept right on hiccuping.

He ran through the whole spectrum of old wives' remedies, trying everything anyone suggested. He stood on his head with his feet propped against the wall as long as he could hold the position. He ran until he was ready to drop from exhaustion. He drank water until he felt like he was drowning. He sucked on a lemon. He had friends and relatives pound him on the back and squeeze him around the middle. Nothing worked.

One day someone told him about Dr. Reder. Seth asked around (still hiccuping) and the whole procedure sounded like absolute nonsense. However, just as most of Dr. Reder's patients have done, he went to the Park Avenue office in an act of pure desperation. He says: "Still hiccuping, I sat down in the chair and permitted Dr. Reder to insert the applicators in my nose. My only sensation was a tear or two as he inserted them. Then I just sat there waiting for my next hiccup.

"The next hiccup never came! I couldn't believe it! But I was still afraid that they would start again when he removed the applicators. After half an hour he began to take them out. I pleaded, 'Dr. Reder, can't we leave them in longer? I'm afraid I'll start to hiccup again.' Dr. Reder laughed at me and said firmly, 'You're not going to start hiccuping again. That's all over with.' And he was right."

I asked, "Are you still coming to Dr. Reder for treatment for hiccups?" "No," he replied, "I come to him for any kind of pain now. I recently suffered from lower back pain, and instead of making the rounds of orthopedic surgeons and neurologists and so on, I decided to come here first. You know what? It works very well. I come about once a week now to control the lower back pain."

"Do you still get hiccup attacks?" I asked.

"I did get one or two attacks after the one that brought me here, and I came right back for further treatments. After a few attacks, I stopped getting them at all. I haven't had a hiccup attack for several years."

Tintinnabulation—I Hear the Bells Ringing

Mary Moran is a school teacher. She was in good health and good spirits until about five years ago when she began to hear a ringing in her ears. When it started, it was very very soft, barely audible, but it gradually got louder.

She visited her family doctor, who sent her to an otolaryngologist. The ear, nose and throat man examined her. He tried washing her ears, but this didn't help at all. "In fact," she told me, "I think after the washing, the ringing got louder."

She continued, "The doctor explained that I had tinnitus. That's just the fancy medical name for ringing in the ears. They really have no treatment for it because they don't know what it is or what causes it. I started to make the rounds of doctors, when my friends urged me to try this one or that one who might be able to help. They all had someone to suggest, but the bottom line was always that they didn't really know what to do.

"At last I concluded that none of the doctors could possibly help me because most of them suspected that it was psychosomatic—I just thought I heard the ringing. I believe that, because they couldn't hear it, they didn't really believe that I could. Well, I did hear it and it interfered with my classroom teaching, it interfered with my entire life."

Like so many other desperate people suffering from a condition which the medical profession could not properly diagnose, treat or cure, she ended up in Dr. Reder's office. She says, "His first treatment didn't work. It may have muffled the ringing a little, but I could still hear those bells and they still were loud enough to annoy me and irritate me."

"But you continued to see Dr. Reder?"

"Oh, I surely did. I figured if it had any effect at all, even making it softer, more treatments might do even better. This was the first treatment that had ever helped even a little bit. Up to that time, the only treatments I got, like cleaning my ears, did me more harm than good. No way would I quit now, when something had at least a faint possibility of helping."

She continued with the treatments every other day for several weeks. "Then," she explained, "I started to feel I was getting some relief out of it. Sometimes, especially immediately after a treatment, the sounds went away completely. It's true that sometimes they came back within a few hours. I did notice that, as I continued the treatments, the intervals of silence, with no bells ringing, got longer and longer. Finally, I got to the point where I went for several months without a spell of tinnitus."

I asked, "How are you now?"

She smiled, "Completely normal. As long as I see Dr. Reder once every other week, I have no tinnitus at all. I haven't heard a bell, except our church bells, for almost a year. And please believe me, I intend to keep it that way."

The Woman Who Had to Go Skiing

Dorothy Dalton was an attractive woman in her early thirties. While I was interviewing various patients, Dorothy had fixed her penetrating eyes on me, a look of curiosity sparkling in them. I had never spoken to her because, as she usually reclined on a couch after her applicators were inserted, I felt I might be disturbing her by requesting an interview. One afternoon while I sat in the lounge organizing my dictating equipment, she approached me and asked, "Aren't you going to interview me?"

I said, "I've been reluctant to disturb you, but I would be delighted if you would give me an interview."

With a broad smile, she answered, "I may have experienced the best miracle of all!"

Dorothy is an athletic woman. She played tennis and racquet ball, and had acquired a degree of expertise on skis. Approximately three years ago she met a man who attracted her. While jogging in Central Park she had literally bumped into him. Thereafter, every morning for several days they passed each other on the jogging track. Ultimately, they fell into conversation, and Dorothy learned that he too enjoyed both tennis and racquet ball. She also discovered he enjoyed skiing.

They dated a few times; they played racquet ball together; early in November, he suggested going to Vermont for a skiing weekend in early December. Up to this time she had been unable to break through the reserve of the shy young man; they had never really become intimate. Nevertheless, she longed to have a closer relationship with him.

She told me frankly, "I have met very few men who inspired me with any desire to sleep with them. However, Charlie really turned me on, and I had a burning desire to find out if he was as good in bed as he was on the court."

Dorothy quickly agreed to the December date. She carefully checked over her skiing equipment, and made sure her clothing was in good order. She was filled with happy anticipation about the weekend in Vermont. Ten days before they were supposed to leave, Dorothy twisted her ankle on the racquet ball court. The doctor who examined her assured her that according to the x-rays, nothing was broken. It was simply a condition that would heal itself.

He called it a "tenosynovitis" and explained, "It's what we call a self-limiting injury. At most, it might last as long as six weeks, but it probably will be completely healed within three weeks."

Dorothy told the doctor anxiously, "I have a skiing date in ten days and I really don't want to have to cancel it. Isn't there anything you can do?"

The doctor said dubiously, "I don't think you should attempt skiing in ten days, even if your ankle feels better. A tenosynovitus is an inflammation of the tendon's sheath. The tendons are fibrous bands which connect muscle to bone. Even though they are quite strong, they can be injured and become inflamed, and that's what happened with your ankle. I doubt if I can give you enough relief to permit skiing in ten days, but I can try a steroid shot. It might speed up healing."

Dorothy really hated to take any chance of missing that

skiing date with Charlie. She knew, of course, she could make the trip even if she couldn't actually ski, but that would spoil all the fun. She had planned to impress Charlie with her competence on skis, and anything less wouldn't satisfy her. But her ankle hurt and would scarcely bear her weight walking, let alone skiing. On the other hand, she was reluctant to risk taking steroids.

Three days before the trip to Vermont Dorothy had a movie date with Charlie. She told Charlie what had happened to her ankle. He listened sympathetically, and suggested, "I know a Dr. Milton Reder. He has offices on Park Avenue and I'd like you to see him. In a situation like yours, he has been known to perform miracles."

When Dorothy heard exactly the kind of therapy Dr. Reder used, she was dubious about whether it could possibly do her any good. However, if it would please Charlie to take her there, she would go. The next afternoon they went for her first Reder treatment.

Dorothy said, "I walked into that office and I couldn't believe my eyes. It struck me as totally absurd. I saw a big room with people sitting around, or standing and talking, completely unconcerned—but everyone had wires sticking out of their noses. Let me tell you, I was completely unimpressed with that scene. I thought to myself, 'There's no way this can do me any good. It's my ankle, not my nose, that's giving me trouble.'"

But Dorothy was already there, and it was all part of pleasing Charlie, so she agreed to at least meet Dr. Reder. Jokingly, she told him, "Charlie and I are supposed to go skiing in Vermont Friday night, for the weekend. Can you make me better by then?"

Dr. Reder answered, "My God, this is only Wednesday and you want to be all better by Friday! I'm glad you didn't wait until Thursday. You're giving me a lot of extra time."

She gave Reder a sheepish glance, then answered the questions he asked her. Seeming satisfied with the answers, the doctor inserted the applicators into her nose.

Dorothy told me, "I saw no possibility that these wires could do any good for my ankle. I felt like I had walked through the Looking Glass, or wandered into a jungle hut where a witch doctor practiced. But Charlie had told me about all kinds of miraculous cures performed by Dr. Reder, and I didn't see any way to walk out right then, so I just sat there with those ridiculous wires sticking out of my nose, feeling like the village idiot.

"Even though I didn't believe it could do any good, I sat quietly waiting for the half hour to pass so I could have them removed. Since I had hurt my ankle, I had gotten into the habit of propping my foot up on something when I sat down, because it relieved the pain. Now, as I sat in Dr. Reder's office, I suddenly realized that both feet were firmly planted on the floor in front of me, and nothing hurt. I pushed down on my right foot, in a way that practically guaranteed a pang. Still nothing hurt."

In spite of the fact that she had been convinced that this treatment would do no good, Dorothy now admitted to the first flutters of hope. She told Dr. Reder, "I'd like to stand up. My ankle feels pretty good, and I'd like to find out if it will hurt when I stand on it."

Dr. Reder smilingly said, "If the treatment can do you any good at all, it will do you a lot of good. Go ahead, get up and see if you can walk on it."

The applicators had now been in Dorothy's nose for about twenty minutes. She stood up, placing her full weight on both feet. She braced herself for the sharp pain she always felt when she did anything like that, but this time nothing hurt. She took a tentative step, supporting her weight on her good left foot. Even this distribution of weight had been causing her pain. This time it felt fine!

Now she stepped forward, placing all her weight on her right foot. To her utter delight, she felt no pain at all.

She said to me, "Incredible as it may sound, all the pain had been removed by that one treatment! I felt sure that I could walk, run, jump, or ski, and my ankle would not hurt. I certainly never expected such a result. To me, this was an authentic miracle."

When I asked if she had gone skiing that weekend, her eyes lit up. She said, "Did I ever! Charlie and I skied all day Saturday, and all-in-all I had the best weekend of my life."

Just to finish up the story, I asked about Charlie. She replied, "Yes, I see him every day. Shortly after that weekend, we got married."

CHAPTER IX

An "Arthritis Expert" and Other Grateful Human Beings

Chester Chait regards himself as the world's leading expert on arthritis. He favored me with a lecture on the subject. "Arthritis is really more than a hundred different kinds of diseases. It affects more than twenty million Americans and can occur in any joint in the body. It could be the toes, the knees, any place along the spinal column, in the finger, the hips, or any other joint. It may interest you to know that I am probably one of the few living people with arthritis in almost every joint. You might say, I'm arthritis-prone."

In addition to normal joint pains, arthritis can also cause fever, loss of appetite, disturbance of vision, and stiffness, especially in weight-bearing joints like the ankles, knees and hips.

Chester has suffered flare-ups of arthritis so severe at times as to require hospitalization. In the hospital they

Indomethacin, Butazolidin, or Prednesone. "However," he adds, "Prednesone is a steroid and must be avoided by me at all times because of the really unpleasant side effects."

Chester went on to say, "I remember once I had such severe pain in my right knee that the doctor suggested I should seriously consider surgical removal of the membrane lining the knee joint."

I asked, "Did you consider it?"

"To tell the truth, I not only considered it, but I was actually scheduled for surgery. I welcomed the idea, because I kept thinking of the blessed relief from pain I would have afterward."

As things worked out, he didn't need the surgery. Following a trail of doctors throughout greater New York City, he finally picked up a reference to Dr. Milton Reder. One afternoon, a few years ago, a desperate Chester arrived at the Park Avenue office. While he gave Dr. Reder his case history, he mentioned that he was scheduled for surgery the following week.

Reder advised him, "My treatment has proved fairly good for arthritis. I can't tell you it's a hundred percent but it has done a lot for many people. I suggest you postpone the surgery and try a few weeks of this treatment. The surgery only has a partial chance of success, anyway, and you can always have it later."

It didn't take much convincing to get Chester to postpone the operation, and he began to take the Reder treatments. He said, "I really didn't believe it would do me any good. But then I met so many people here with so many kinds of aches and pains, including those with arthritis, that I couldn't help listening. Many of them told me they had experienced prompt relief after taking the Reder treatment.

"Well, the first treatment I got hardly even dented the

pain. It's true that my pain was firmly entrenched in my body by then, and I didn't expect any miracles. But the stories of other patients did encourage me, so I hung in. In the beginning, I came every day, and on some days I took two treatments.

"After two weeks I realized that my pain was diminishing. I could sleep several consecutive hours each night, instead of waking up in pain every time I moved. I could watch television for as much as fifteen or twenty minutes at a stretch without having to get up and walk around. I also went for increasing periods of time without taking pain killers, and I eventually got through an entire day without taking even an aspirin."

After three months of regular treatment, Chester Chait, for the first time in many years, became completely free of pain. He told me, "No one who has not experienced being in constant pain month after month, and year after year, every minute of the day can appreciate what it means to be completely pain-free. Even though it took many months to achieve this, it was worth every minute I spent sitting in Reder's office, just to reach this final pinnacle of a pain-free body."

"How often do you have to get the treatments now," I asked, "in order to stay free of pain?"

"Well, it varies a good bit, depending on my activity. If I'm physically active, walking around, and doing the exercises my physical therapist prescribes, I get away with just one weekly treatment. But if I get too involved with my work, and I stop doing my exercises, then I have to come more frequently. I can always tell in advance, because I start to get warning twinges, and then I rush to Dr. Reder's office for treatment.

"As soon as I feel the onset of pain, I take one, or even two, treatments a day until I stop hurting again. I've had enough experience with this pain so I can tell when it needs frequent treatment, and when I can go back to the once-a-week routine. Sometimes I can even get it down to once every other week. I know it may sound like a hassle to have to come here so frequently, but believe me, feeling like a human being again is worth anything."

SGB vs. Open Heart Surgery

Dr. Harry Hardesty is Chief of Pediatrics in a New York hospital. When Dr. Hardesty began to experience chest pains which radiated down his left arm, he knew at once that he had a classic case of angina pectoris, but he refused to accept it. Even so, he maintained a careful watch over his vital signs.

He learned that if he walked rapidly, he had chest pains. If he stopped and rested, the pain disappeared. If he went out in cold weather, the pain started, and it left when he went inside and sat down.

He told me, "It was obvious to me that I had atherosclerosis. This caused my coronary arteries to narrow and reduced the blood supply to my heart. Exercise increases the heart beat, causing the heart muscle to need more blood flow and, because of the narrowed passage, pain results. When I reduce my activities, the blood flow becomes adequate to supply my heart and the pain stops."

Dr. Hardesty knew that angina is a serious disorder, because its presence clearly denotes diseased coronary arteries. He realized he needed treatment. Finally he went to the most esteemed cardiologist in his hospital, had a complete examination that included an electro-cardiogram, and then got instructions from the cardiologist on future behavior. These included the need to take off twenty pounds, to stop smoking, and to stay away from smokers and smoky places, and to eliminate fat almost completely from his diet. The cardiologist also prescribed glyceryl trinitrate (nitro-glycerine) caps with instructions to place one under his tongue if he felt severe pain. The cap would dissolve, enter the bloodstream, and dilate the coronary arteries. This would eliminate the pain. He had to avoid heavy exercise, and substitute mild calesthenics.

Finally, the cardiologist said, "Let's try this regimen to begin with. Later we can see if we need any beta-adrenegic blocking agents."

Dr. Hardesty followed the cardiologist's advice religiously. He went on a diet and lost twenty-five pounds. He gave up smoking completely, and avoided all foods containing cholesterol.

For a while the new regimen worked, and, although he still got angina pain if he walked too fast or did anything else to cause a rapid heart beat, he could live with the condition. As time went by, however, the severe pain recurred. At first it was occasional, then more frequent, and finally he had pain most of the time.

When I interviewed him, the doctor explained to me, "You see, in atherosclerosis, fatty deposits accumulate and harden on the arterial walls, forming scar-like patches. Sometimes these are called intimas or plaques. They form gradually in the coronary arteries that provide the heart with its vital blood supply. Once the plaques form, they become natural lodging places for other deposits like fat, calcium, and even blood clots. Eventually the plaques start to fill up the channel of the artery, like lime forming in a pipe, and this stops the flow of blood. Any time the heart muscle doesn't get enough blood to do its work, chest pains result. That was what I suffered from."

When the pain became constant, Dr. Hardesty went back to his cardiologist for further treatment. The cardiologist tried more heroic measures, but the pain persisted. At last he told Hardesty, "I have the feeling that your circulation is not as bad as the pain seems to indicate.

Some people seem to have a lower tolerance for pain. You may be in that class. Most of the indications I see are that your circulation is adequate, and that your arteries are in fairly good health. Even so, if you want something more definitive, we'll have to go in surgically and do a by-pass."

Dr. Hardesty continued, "By-pass surgery involves taking an artery from another part of the body, where it can be spared, and using it to replace the diseased artery by grafting it in place. This procedure bypasses the occluded coronary artery.

"Many laymen will accept the by-pass surgery. It sounds logical, and it's performed regularly, with reasonable success. But we physicians frequently know too much. For example, some years ago there was a surgical procedure for handling my problem, where blood from other vessels was diverted to the heart. The operation was touted as giving great benefit in the relief of pain. Then a controlled study was done. Half the candidates for the procedure had the full surgical procedure performed, while the other half had the chest opened and closed, with no other surgery taking place. All patients were told that the surgery had taken place. The results insofar as relief of pain was concerned, were exactly the same in both groups!"

[For those interested in this topic, I want to mention that I located a reference to that study in a book by Steven F. Brena, M.D., entitled *Chronic Pain, America's Hidden Epidemic* (New York: Atheneum, 1978), page 51.]

Dr. Hardesty remained unconvinced that bypass surgery was the answer to his problem. He searched for alternate solutions. While talking to one of his own patients, he learned about Dr. Reder. The patient, a sixteen-year-old boy, had been in an accident. While riding his bicycle, he was hit by an automobile, and he struck his elbow a very hard blow. This produced constant, unremitting pain. Dr. Hardesty had tried unsuccessfully to treat it, and then referred him to a rheumatologist. One day the boy came back to Hardesty with another problem and Hardesty asked about the elbow pain. His patient told him that the rheumatologist had referred him to Dr. Milton Reder, and he spoke with enthusiasm about how Dr. Reder had relieved his pain.

The pain of angina continued to trouble Dr. Hardesty, and he couldn't forget what his young patient had told him about Dr. Reder. Finally he decided to check it out, and to try the, to him, bizarre treatment.

He conferred with Dr. Reder, who told him, "The sphenopalatine ganglion blockade has at times given some success in exactly such cases as yours. I don't really know why it works, except that it does tend to lower blood pressure. I've had a number of experiences with patients where angina pain has either been reduced or eliminated with SGB."

"I had very little hope," Dr. Hardesty said to me, "but I was desperate, so I told him to go ahead with the treatment."

At the time he received the first treatment, Dr. Hardesty was not suffering any pain. After an hour, when Dr. Reder removed the applicators, Hardesty remarked, "Well, I've had the treatment, now how will I know if it does me any good?"

Reder replied, "I tell you what—you go out and take a walk around the block. I'm sure if you walk at all rapidly, you'll feel the angina pain. Go see how bad it gets, and then come back and tell me."

Hardesty took Reder's advice, and went for a brisk walk. Tentatively, he increased his pace and he did feel some pain, but not as severe as he had feared. He reported back to Reder, who smiled at him and said, "One good thing about this treatment is that if it has any effect at all, it is highly effective. I know very early with each person if it will be any use to continue. In your case, I predict that if you stay with it, you'll have a lot of relief."

Dr. Hardesty reported to 555 Park Avenue every day for two weeks for treatment. He said, "At the end of the fourteenth treatment, I was completely free of angina pain, unless I indulged in very rigorous exercise. I could enjoy all of my normal, accustomed activities, including walking a few blocks at a reasonable pace, walking up a flight of steps, and doing a lot of other things that would have produced severe angina pain before I started treatment with Dr. Reder."

Dr. Hardesty still visits Dr. Reder for treatment once or twice a week, but he no longer suffers from angina pain, and he didn't have to have bypass surgery to get rid of it.

The Blink That Hurts

Mrs. Myra Mueller is a gray-haired woman in her early sixties with a ramrod back. When I asked her why she came to see Dr. Reder, she replied brusquely, "I have a corneal abrasion in my right eye. I woke up one morning and every time I blinked I felt a sharp pain in my head."

She immediately visited her opthalmologist, who gave her a careful examination and diagnosed a corneal abrasion. He prescribed some drops to use several times a day, and assured her the abrasion would heal with no after effects. In spite of his assurances, in actual fact her eye condition deteriorated. Every time she blinked, she could feel the sharp pain, and it became increasingly annoying.

She started to make the rounds of eye specialists. They all said, "You have a corneal abrasion." They had no problem making the diagnosis, but no one could heal the condition. Each doctor gave her a different kind of drops, but nothing did any good. Her suffering continued every time her eye blinked.

Mrs. Mueller's husband was a patient of Dr. Reder, who was treating him for a back problem. He urged her to try the Reder treatment. She had been in Reder's office with her husband on occasion, and she had a very low opinion of the treatment.

She remarked to me, "It struck me as the height of absurdity to see all these otherwise normal people sitting around with wires stuck up their noses, just as though that could cure anybody of anything. I was sure that any cure they experienced had to be psychosomatic."

In desperation she finally did consult Dr. Reder, and told him about her corneal abrasion. Dr. Reder told her dubiously, "I frankly don't know. I don't think I've ever treated such a case as yours. However," Dr. Reder challenged, "let's give it a try and, if it doesn't work, you don't have to pay me."

Mrs. Mueller continued, "I took the treatment with not the slightest expectation that it could possibly help me. My husband had already told me that the applicators didn't hurt when they were inserted, so I was completely relaxed. Dr. Reder told me to sit quietly and just rest. I did just that. Naturally, while I was sitting there, I did blink occasionally and it hurt. Then, to my surprise, after about ten or fifteen minutes, I became aware that the pain which came with each blink had started to ease. Incredible as it might sound, in another ten minutes the pain was completely gone!"

I asked Mrs. Mueller, "Do you still come to see Dr. Reder for the corneal pain?"

"No," she replied, "that problem disappeared more than a year ago. As I understand it, it was the relief of pain which allowed the eye to heal itself. After nine or ten treatments, spread out over a few weeks, the cornea itself started to heal. In fact, I went back to my ophthalmologist a few months after I saw doctor Reder, and had my eye examined. He said the abrasion was completely healed."

She continued, "I come now occasionally for other pain. Right now I have a lower back pain which comes back from time to time."

I asked, "Could any of the eye doctors you saw explain why the sphenopalatine ganglion blockade works to either stop the pain, or heal, an abraded cornea?"

She answered, "Well, one of the doctors told me that in his opinion it was like taking an aspirin."

Mrs. Mueller continued, "You know, when you have a headache and you take an aspirin or a Tylenol, it deadens the pain, but it also does more than that. It allows the body to adjust itself so that the headache disappears. People frequently ask me how long Dr. Reder's treatment works, and I think of it in the same way as an aspirin or Tylenol. When you take the aspirin for a headache, you really get rid of the headache, and when the aspirin wears off, the headache usually doesn't come back because it's gone out of the body. As I see it, the Reder treatment works in a similar way. The SGB eliminated the pain when I blinked, and, with the pain gone, my body could take over and start to heal the cause of the pain. So the SGB and my body worked together to heal my corneal abrasion."

I guess this is as good a theory as any I have heard to explain the phenomenonal results obtained by the SGB.

The Tummyache That Wouldn't Go Away

Albert Adelman is a short, roly-poly man in his middle sixties. His twinkling eye and hearty laugh invited me to join him in some private joke. When I approached him for an interview, and asked my usual question, "Why are you here in Dr. Reder's office?" he replied, "I came the first time because I had a tummyache that wouldn't go away."

In questioning him further, the following story emerged: Mr. Adelman led a healthy life, rarely suffering from anything that might cause him pain. He visited his doctor once a year, and he visited his dentist twice a year. His health was completely satisfactory. Then, one day at about ten o'clock in the morning, he suddenly got a stomach ache. It wasn't very severe, but he did feel some pain in the lower part of his abdomen toward the left side. At times he felt as though he had to move his bowels, but it was usually a false alarm. About the pain, however, there was no doubt. Usually about an hour after it started, it would disappear, but it would come back the next day at about the same time. This annoyed Mr. Adelman no end, so he made an appointment to see his physician.

Dr. Smith listened carefully to his complaint, and gave him a thorough examination. He palpated the area in question with his fingertips, and then used his stethoscope to listen to various parts of the body, especially trying to auscultate the bowel area.

When he completed the examination, Dr. Smith told Albert Adelman, "I'm afraid we'll have to send you in for a barium x-ray. This is the only way I can make a definitive diagnosis."

Later Mr. Adelman learned that Dr. Smith was afraid of a possible malignant tumor somewhere in the lower intestine. However, until he was certain of his diagnosis, he saw no point in worrying his patient, so he said nothing.

Albert Adelman dutifully swallowed the barium and stretched out on the table while the technicians took x-ray after x-ray of his lower intestinal area.

Luckily for Albert, the x-rays were negative. What it did show was some diverticula (small pouches which form on the walls of the large intestine). Dr. Smith explained to his anxious patient, "Sometimes these diverticula become inflamed. That's what we call diverticulitis."

Albert asked, "So what you are saying is that I have a condition called 'diverticulitis,' right?"

"Exactly," said Dr. Smith. "In itself, diverticulitis is not a very serious condition. It's always possible that it might become serious if you should have an acute attack. Then you would have a lot of pain and tenderness in the lower abdominal area, and you would also probably run a temperature. However, I doubt if you have anything to worry about. There's probably just a little inflammation on one of the diverticula, and that's causing the pain. Now, if you follow the diet I'm giving you, I feel sure the inflammation will clear up."

Mr. Adelman followed the doctor's orders meticulously, but the bellyache kept coming back. Sometimes it came back at ten in the morning and sometimes it waited until two in the afternoon, but come back it did. He went back to Dr. Smith, who checked him out very carefully.

The doctor reported, "You seem to be in excellent health. All your vital signs are good and I find very little reason for you to have these stomachaches. If you had a severe attack of diverticulitis, I'm sure you would have much more tenderness in the lower abdomen. And you would also probably have fever. But you don't have any of these symptoms. I'm telling you, Albert, you have nothing serious to worry about."

"But, doctor," Adelman protested, "I keep having these pains. They're interfering with my work."

Dr. Smith suggested pain killers, starting with aspirin or Tylenol. If that didn't do the job, he would give him a prescription for something stronger. Adelman, however, was not satisfied with such treatment.

"Dr. Smith," he said, "I'm an advertising copywriter. I have to be alert all the time. I know from past experience that if I take a pain killer of any kind, I might just as well not go to work that day. I lose all my creativity when I'm fuzzy from pain killers. I can't write if I can't think straight. Even if I just get a back headache I have to either suffer, or take a pill and give up work for the rest of the day."

The doctor shrugged his shoulders and said, "Maybe you should see a gastroenterologist. I suggest you see Dr. Johnson. He's a good man and might be able to help you."

Dr. Johnson confirmed Dr. Smith's diagnosis. He told Adelman, "I have no doubt that you're suffering from inflammation of the diverticula. However, I feel sure I can help you. The pain will definitely go away if you're just patient."

Albert Adelman was not a patient man, and it was not in his nature just to sit around and wait for improvement. His condition interfered with his creativity, whether he just bore the pain stoically or took pain killers. As happened to so many people, so it happened to Mr. Adelman. Someone told him about Milton Reder, and suggested he visit that doctor.

In desperation, ready to try anything by now, Adelman went to 555 Park Avenue. He didn't really expect cocaine-dipped applicators in his nose to help his diverticulitis, but to his complete amazement he discovered that his attacks diminished, and finally stopped altogether.

Now he worried that the elimination of the pain only masked symptoms, rather than offering the hope of a cure. He was afraid that sooner or later he would have a severe attack which at worst might end in a perforation and result in peritonitis. He had done enough reading on the subject of diverticulitis to know this was a distinct possibility. So back he went to Dr. Johnson.

Johnson listened incredulously to Adelman's story. Finally he said, "What you're saying makes absolutely no sense. I never heard of such nonsense. The fact that the anesthetization of a small ganglion in your head could possibly cure a stomachache is beyond belief. On the other hand, if you don't have stomachaches any more, then don't worry about inflammation or perforation or peritonitis. Just forget the whole thing. I'd like you to come back in six months for a checkup, and we'll watch carefully to be sure that the condition has in fact cleared up."

As Adelman finished telling me his story, he laughed and commented, "I sure wish Dr. Reder would let me advertise him. I could write the best copy the world has every read. But when I suggest it to him he just laughs at me. He says he's got more than enough patients for an octogenarian physician."

CHAPTER X

Do You Know You Have a Tunnel In Your Wrist?

Harriet Hopkins is a school teacher in her late twenties or early thirties. She tends to carry her school teacher mannerisms with her when she leaves school. When I asked her what brought her to 555 Park Avenue, she replied with another question, "Did you know you have a tunnel in your wrist?"

I admitted my ignorance. Harriet lectured, "Well, the tendons in your wrist pass through a tunnel, together with a large nerve, the median, which also passes through the same tunnel. Lots of people, especially women, suffer from certain symptoms, including numbness, tingling, and burning pain in the entire hand. The pain spreads through the whole area to which the median nerve supplies sensation. That includes the thumb, the index finger, the middle finger and a small part of the ring finger."

Harriet Hopkins first felt these sensations one night when she was awakened by a painful tingling. The pain persisted at night, and then invaded her days too. After a while it began to interfere with her ability to teach.

Her doctor explained, "Yours is a common condition called 'carpal tunnel syndrome,' which attacks a large number of people. Women seem to suffer from it more than men."

In the beginning, the doctor gave Harriet a removable splint with instructions to wear it at night, and whenever her hand hurt. She used the splint for a week with little relief, so she went back to the doctor, who gave her an injection of cortisone.

She experienced some relief for a few days, and then the pain returned. She worried about becoming steroid dependent, so she looked around for another doctor.

A friend suggested the name of a doctor who was a wrist specialist. This doctor was reputed to be expert in carpal tunnel syndrome. He listened to her symptoms, examined her carefully, and recommended surgery.

"This type of surgery is relatively minor," he explained, "and it will reduce the pressure in the tunnel. What we do is to divide the ligaments which lie above the tunnel."

Harriet Hopkins would not use steroids, and she wouldn't allow surgery! Her father had died on the operating table during "routine" heart surgery. The mere thought of an operating room terrified her. She lived with her pain for a while and then, about a year before our conversation took place, she read an article in *New York* magazine. She told me, "The article was quite pejorative. The writer spoke of Dr. Milton Reder in a very deprecating way, and made it clear he thought very little of him and his treatments. However, in reading between the lines, I concluded that Dr. Reder's treatment was rather unusual and maybe it could help me. I decided that, in spite of the unflattering article, I would see this doctor."

Harriet Hopkins arrived at Reder's office with a completely neutral attitude. She had high hopes, and a lot of interest in what was going on there, but she approached the treatment cautiously, waiting to see what would happen before she formed an opinion about its efficacy.

She described her first visit to me. "I sat down in that chair and let him insert the wires into my nose. He assured me that it wouldn't hurt, although it might bring a tear or two to my eyes. He made no promises. When I asked him if the treatment would help the carpal tunnel syndrome pain, he said only, 'Let's wait and see.'"

Harriet took the treatment and, although at that time she had no real wrist pain, she could feel her wrist relax in a way it had not until then. For the next several hours she felt no pain at all, but during the night the pain returned fleetingly. But she did get enough relief to convince her to try another treatment. The next afternoon she was back in the Park Avenue office for her second treatment. It was the first time in a year that she had been pain-free for twenty-four hours.

She told me softly, "The most blessed thing about it was that I slept through an entire night without that fiendish pain in my wrist waking me."

Many activies were going on in her life at the time, so she went for three days without treatment, after which the pain returned. After that she made it a point to visit Dr. Reder every day for the next two weeks. Then Dr. Reder suggested she come only every other day. A month later, she cut back to every third day.

I asked, "Are you still here for treatment of the carpal tunnel syndrome?"

"Yes, that's right. That's what I'm here for now. But now I only have to come once every few weeks. I don't really know if I have to come at all, because I haven't had an attack in several months. I just feel more comfortable if I get a treatment from time to time just to be sure the pain won't come back. I guess I'm afraid to find out if I could do without them altogether."

Dr. Milton Reder vs. Sir Charles Bell

Mary Martino is a tall, slender and very attractive young woman with soft blond hair and fair skin. Her winning smile lights her face in charming fashion. It did not surprise me to learn that she is a member of the cast of a long-running CBS afternoon TV soap opera.

One morning she woke from a deep sleep with a sensation of numbness in her face. She went to the bathroom and looked into the mirror. Horrified, she saw that one side of her face was, in her own language, "askew. The left side of my face was all lopsided. It was awful. And what was even worse was that I couldn't go to work looking like that. I couldn't even let anyone see me. I had to do something! And fast!"

She dressed as quickly as she could and hurried to her physician. Fortunately for her, he was in the office and saw her immediately. After examining her, he pronounced, "You have Bell's Palsy, I'm afraid. It's a form of paralysis of the facial nerves. Because it happened only on one side, it gives the lopsided appearance."

Noting her shocked expression, he continued reassuringly, "It comes without warning, and recovery will be spontaneous. You should begin to recover within a week. Generally speaking, recovery is complete within several weeks from onset."

That prognosis might be okay for most people, but an actress dependent on her appearance, and working in a daily TV show, didn't have several weeks to wait. The occurrence took place on Friday, and she was due on the set Monday.

"I could probably have arranged to be written out of the episode which was shooting that Monday," she said, "and I probably could have gotten off for as long as a week. But I couldn't stretch it any further, and I certainly didn't want to take a chance on being written out altogether. Also, to tell the truth, I was afraid to show up on the set and have them see me like that. Who knows what might happen?"

Frantically, she pressed her doctor, but he could offer no promise of any quicker relief. That was the timetable for Bell's Palsy and it couldn't be changed.

She told me, "I'm a researcher from way back. I was a science major in college, and I supported myself for two years doing research for a magazine. I immediately went to the New York Academy of Medicine Library to do research on Bell's Palsy. I learned that, as the doctor had told me, it was a paralysis of the facial nerve. In my case the paralysis was of unknown origin. I learned that the condition had first been described in 1828 by Sir Charles Bell, a Scottish surgeon. I also read a confirmation of what the doctor had said: healing would begin from a week to a few weeks after the onset of the attack."

Disheartened, she returned to her apartment. She telephoned her friends for any suggestions they might have. "I told everybody I spoke with that I needed a miracle."

One friend said, "Mary, I think I should tell you about Dr. Milton Reder. He's at 555 Park Avenue. Go to see him. I know of one miracle he performed for someone who suffered from migraine. Maybe he can help."

When Mary discovered that Dr. Reder had ongoing office hours and required no appointment, she took a cab over at once. Seated opposite Dr. Reder, she asked, "Can your treatment help Bell's Palsy?"

Dr. Reder told her, "Yes, I've had cases where it worked very well, and others where it does nothing. Let's give it a try."

"What I need to know right now," she said, "is, can the treatment make it worse?"

He answered in true Reder fashion, "It will help, or it won't help, but it won't make it worse. Don't worry."

She took her first treatment at about eleven A.M. on Friday. After the applicators had been inserted, she went into the bathroom to check her face. She said, "I may have been kidding myself, but when I examined my face carefully, it seemed to me that it was just a little less lopsided than it had been when I arrived."

She returned to Dr. Reder's office and said, "Doctor, I really think that your treatment has helped a little already. I'd like to have as many treatments as possible between now and Monday. Maybe I'll really be able to report to the set on schedule."

"Well," Dr. Reder replied, "you can have two treatments a day, but that's the limit. I'll be here Saturday and Sunday, so you come in then."

She hung around the office that Friday to receive a second treatment. Saturday she was in the office by eight o'clock for her first insertions, and came back again at three for another set. Sunday she repeated this schedule.

"What happened then?" I asked.

"By Sunday evening my face was almost completely normal. There was just a trace of a twist left, but not so anybody would notice. I could face the cameras. I continued my visits to Dr. Reder. He'd saved my job!"

After three weeks of daily treatments, the Bell's Palsy was gone completely. "Believe me," she said earnestly, "I scrutinized my face minutely under a bright light every day, but I could see no trace of any paralysis."

I asked, "Are you still visiting Dr. Reder for the Bell's Palsy?"

"No," she laughed, "What happened was that I fell recently and hurt my knee. I come now for the pain in my knee so I can walk without it hurting. The Bell's Palsy is long gone, thanks to Dr. Reder."

"He Keeps My Father Alive"

Linda Lavery is a 25-year-old nurse who works in a New York hospital. To look at her no one would believe that she needed Reder therapy for anything. I noticed her sitting on one of the couches at Dr. Reder's because she was one of the few people in the room without applicators in her nose. By now I had spent a lot of time in Dr. Reder's office, and felt like an old hand.

I approached her. "Are you a patient, or a 'bringer of patient,' " I asked her.

My question brought a smile to her lips. She answered, "I guess you could call me a 'bringer.' "

I learned that she came once a week to bring her father, John Lavery, for the Reder treatment. She said, "My father has the Adams-Stokes syndrome. It's something that affects primarily older people."

The syndrome was discovered when Mr. Lavery, while taking his accustomed nap after dinner, couldn't be awakened. His family found that he was unconscious, not sleeping. Assuming that he had had a heart attack, a stroke, or something similar, they called the paramedics, who took him to the hospital. John Lavery was hospitalized for three days, after which he was sent home, diagnosed as a victim of the Adams-Stokes syndrome.

I said, "Linda, I never heard of this syndrome, so could you tell me what it is?"

She explained, "It comes from a disturbance in the heart rhythm. In effect, it's a temporary interruption of the heart beat. If the heart stops beating for anywhere from four to eight seconds, unconsciousness results, especially if the person is standing or sitting erect.

The interruption of the heart beat is called 'asystole' and an asystole which lasts more than twelve seconds, even if the person is lying down, will also cause unconsciousness. An asystole of several minutes leads to cyanosis with complete neurological impairment, and probably death."

The medical team told the Lavery family that there was no known treatment for the Adams-Stokes syndrome, but it could be broken up by the implantation of a pacemaker. At the time, Mr. Lavery was in his middle eighties and the family felt he was not a good candidate for a pacemaker.

Linda was already a registered nurse, working private duty from a nurses' registry. On several of her cases, she had heard references to Dr. Reder. Her informants told her he could treat anything that happened to the human body, especially problems which other physicians couldn't solve.

Her scientific background, acquired during her nurse's training, made her very skeptical. However, she felt pressured to try anything that might help her father. After her father suffered a second attack of the syndrome, she brought him to Dr. Reder's office.

Dr. Reder questioned both John and Linda, and then said, "I don't recall ever having treated anyone for the Adams-Stokes syndrome. But I've learned you never can tell, and I know at least the treatment won't do any harm. We'll try it and see what happens."

Linda concluded, "After his first treatment, my father told me he felt no results. I took him home. We had all been watching him very carefully, but we didn't know what to do about the nights, because we wouldn't be able to tell if he had an attack in his sleep. We were really afraid that if that happened, we would find him dead in the morning.

"I decided that, as long as the treatment obviously did him no harm, I would take him back the next day. From then on, I brought him to Dr. Reder every other day for a few weeks. During this period of time, he didn't have a single attack. We watched him carefully while he napped, and detected no sign of a recurrence of the Adams-Stokes syndrome. Then I cut the visits back to twice a week, and, finally I now bring him in once a week. He has not had a single attack since he started coming here, and, believe me, the whole family is greatly relieved about it."

I asked, "Have you said anything about this therapy to those doctors who treated him for Adams-Stokes?"

She answered, "You bet, I certainly did. In fact, I made a point of it. But, you know, doctors are hard to convince about something they didn't learn in medical school.

The Rabbi With Clergyman's Throat

Rabbi Leonard Levy is a tall, imposing man in his middle fifties. When I approached him for an interview, he spoke freely, although his resonant voice had a slightly hoarse quality to it. He told me, "A few years ago I began to suffer from chorditis. Do you know what that is?"

I shook my head, and waited for an explanation.

"The vocal chords have small fibrous nodules on their surface, and sometimes the nodules become irritated and inflamed. In some cases, the inflammation extends to the membranes of the larynx, in which the vocal chords are housed. That's called chorditis."

"Is the condition painful?" I asked.

"Well, it's really more annoying than painful. It causes

hoarseness and some pain in swallowing. If it gets very bad, it can even make breathing painful." After a short pause, he continued, "Do you know what the popular name for chorditis is?"

Again, I shook my head, and waited expectantly.

"Well, the popular name is 'clergyman's throat' and, although anybody who uses the voice a lot can be a victim of chorditis, it seems most especially to affect clergymen."

Rabbi Levy had been suffering from chorditis off and on for many years. Generally speaking, the problem had not been too serious, because when it happened, he simply rested his voice for a week or two and it would be okay again. Complete voice rest always served to relieve the inflammation. Two years before, he had had an attack of chorditis just about a week before the beginning of the High Holy Days of Rosh Hashona and Yom Kippur. He could hardly consider absenting himself from the pulpit on the holiest days of the year. That juxtaposition of events forced him to search for some cure that would work faster than the usual extended period of complete voice rest.

A member of his congregation told him about a doctor who had given him relief from chronic migraine attacks, so he phoned and got Dr. Reder's address. "I went to Dr. Reder and told him my problem. Dr. Reder's reaction was one more of amusement than concern. He kept joking with me, saying, 'Well, I've found that the sphenopalatine ganglion blockade has often performed miracles in helping people in their pursuit of the devil. I should think it would certainly do as well in God's work.' After a few remarks like that, he gave me the treatment and I rested in that chair," pointing to one, "for the next half hour."

The rapid relief from hoarseness caused Rabbi Levy to become very excited over the prospect of a return to normalcy without the usual prolonged period of silence. He asked, "How often can I take these treatments?"

Reder informed him, as usual, that he could have two a day if that's what he wanted. Rabbi Levy came back the same afternoon for his second treatment, and continued thereafter on a twice-a-day basis until the night before the first high holy day. He took a total of twelve treatments. By that time his voice had returned to normal and he mounted the pulpit on the first evening of Rosh Hashona, his heart full of gratitude as his voice rang out over the congregation.

CHAPTER XI

The Peripheral Benefits, or An Example of Serendipity

In many of my interviews with Dr. Reder's patients, I detected a recurrent thread. In brief, quite a few of them come for treatment of one condition and find that another is unexpectedly benefited. Dr. Reder calls it "peripheral advantages," and one English teacher who told me her story called it a case of serendipity. My own experience is an excellent example of what can happen.

I originally went to see Dr. Reder because of heaviness and pain in my legs between my knees and my ankles which prevented me from playing tennis and other sports. One day one of my tennis partners heard the noted author-humorist David Brenner on Cable TV Health News, telling of a similar problem which bothered him. He said he had obtained relief from Dr. Milton Reder's sphenopalatine ganglion blockade. A little research provided me with Dr. Reder's address, and I went to New York to visit him.

I informed him that my condition had been positively diagnosed by medical "experts" as a case of spinal stenosis.

(Many examinations later, I learned from other medical experts that that diagnosis was incorrect.) Reder was thoroughly familiar with the condition, because he suffers from it himself. This was the first time I heard his famous "let's give it a try."

I took a number of treatments, and, frankly, I couldn't detect any improvement. Of course, I must admit that my wife, my children and my associates all commented that I seemed to be walking much better, and that I appeared to be in much better condition than before the SGB. However, I myself didn't perceive any change.

I had been suffering for several years with arthritis in my right wrist. My physician called it "use arthritis" and attributed it to my tennis and softball. The wrist annoyed me, but I always carried a wrist band, so when the pain became severe I could put on the band and get enough relief to carry on with my normal activities without experiencing any real problem. I never sought treatment for it.

When I went to see Dr. Reder I had been having pain in my wrist, and I wore my wrist band. Later I became aware that my wrist had stopped hurting. Since this had happened to me in the past, I just assumed it to be the end of a self-limiting pain. My wrist pain had never been constant, but it did recur from time to time. On the other hand, I was rarely without the pain for a period of more than a week. This time I observed that the pain did not return even after several weeks. As I dictate this chapter, I calculate my wrist has not bothered me for more than three months, and previously it was many years since I had been free of wrist pain for more than a few days.

The Cure of a Wryneck

The English teacher I mentioned earlier told me this story: She suffered from sciatic pain in her right leg, and as time went on it became more severe. She went to orthopedic physicians and rheumatologists, but they couldn't relieve her of her pain. They suggested vaguely that surgery might help, but she rejected that idea. She had heard too many tales of the problems surgery could cause.

Someone told her about Dr. Reder and, one day, in desperation, she decided to take a chance with him. His treatment sounded too fantastic to be true, but she had nowhere left to go.

The Reder treatments didn't seem to give her much relief from her sciatic pain, but she had also suffered for many years with a condition called torticollis, or wryneck. This is a contraction of the sternocleidomastoid muscle, usually only on one side, resulting in an abnormal position of the head.

She explained: "While it didn't cause me a lot of pain, it did cause me to keep my head tilted. When the muscle contracts, it causes the head to swing over, and therefore I was always going around with my head tilted slightly to the right side. I found this very annoying because my perspective was always askew and people kept asking me what was wrong. I tried many doctors, but none had helped.

"Much to my surprise, Dr. Reder's treatments began to straighten out my head, and I have not had torticollis since I started to visit him. I can feel it coming back, at times, and when that happens I immediately go to Dr. Reder, take a treatment, and the incipient torticollis goes away."

I asked, "How did you make out with the sciatic pain?"

She replied, "I don't think the treatments did that much good for the sciatic pain. Nevertheless, it does go away and stay away from time to time, even at times for as long as a few months. When it returns, I take pain killers and live with it. I don't take the Reder treatment for my sciatica."

The Man Who Couldn't Breathe

Nick Nordstrom, in his early sixties, is balding, somewhat fleshy, and walks with a pronounced stoop. He has suffered from asthma for more than forty years. Statistics indicate that about one percent of the population of the United States suffers from this breathing disorder.

An asthma attack can be brought on when the air passages become obstructed by contraction of the bronchial muscle caused by allergies, infection of the bronchial cells, some form of irritation, such as being exposed to smoke, or even by emotional stress. The result is a severe shortage of breath, frequently a dry cough, wheezing and other respiratory problems.

Nick told me, "Just walking into a room where people have been smoking will bring on an asthma attack. Sometimes the attack is so severe I have had to be rushed to the hospital for emergency treatment."

Nick liked to talk about his asthma, and over the years he had become an expert on the topic. He said, "Dozens of kinds of medicines have been developed to control it. There are sympathomimetic agents such as Epinephrine, Isoproterenol or Terbutaline which are either injected into the blood stream or inhaled. Unfortunately, these have undesirable side effects. They produce a tremor, frequently a headache, and hypertension."

He continued to lecture me. "There are methylxanthines, such as Theophyloine or Aminophyloine. These are taken either orally from a spoon or by means of a rectal suppository. Next there are the corticosteroids, such as Prednisone, which should be avoided at all costs because the side effects are peptic ulcer, rapid weight gain and, frequently, high blood pressure. Finally, of course, there are antibiotics and expectorants."

Nick Nordstrom had run the gamut of all the medicines

in his four decades of struggling with asthma. One day, about five years ago, Nick was involved in an automobile accident. He was driving along, minding his own business (as he put it) when somebody rear-ended him with great force. Nick's head snapped back and he suffered a severe whiplash injury. He developed a chronic pain in the back of his neck which, when left uncared for, produced a very severe headache.

Nick made the usual circuit of medical practitioners: orthopedists and rheumatologists, chiropractors, acupuncturists, and assorted purveyors of exotic pain-relief therapy. Nothing worked. As has happened to so many sufferers, one day someone told him about Dr. Reder and he decided to see him. He felt he no longer had anything much to lose and everything to gain.

At the time of his first visit, he was also suffering from intermittent attacks of asthma. He thought the asthma attacks might have been precipitated by the whiplash injury, but he had suffered from asthma for so many years he tended to ignore the causes and merely took the current medicines. They seemed to be doing him some good, and he didn't really expect anything more. So, ignoring the asthma, he concentrated on getting relief for the pain in his neck.

Dr. Reder began treatment, and Nick experienced almost immediate relief. In addition, to his great surprise his asthma suddenly came under control. He discussed it with Dr. Reder, who told him, "Yes, our sphenopalatine ganglion blockade definitely helps most people who suffer with asthma. It's not an absolute, because success depends somewhat on the causes of the asthma attack. However, the treatment helps almost every kind of muscle spasm, and an asthma attack is the result of a form of muscle spasm."

Nick concluded our interview with this comment: "I

have now, for the first time in forty years, enjoyed several years of respite from my asthma attacks. As long as I come in for a treatment twice a week, I don't have any asthma attacks. I can't explain it; I just don't have attacks any more. I have no question in my mind that Dr. Reder's treatment definitely controls my asthma."

The Blockade vs. a Herpes Attack

I interviewed an elderly male patient, who told me the following story:

"I've been coming to see Dr. Milton Reder off and on for the past ten years. I'm subject to lumbo-sacral pain, and when it flares up, I come for a treatment. Sometimes it takes two or three treatments, and sometimes I have to come every day for a week. However, my pain is almost always relieved within that time. Then I can usually stay away for a month or two, and even sometimes as long as three months.

"Three months ago I experienced a flareup of my lumbo-sacral pain, and almost simultaneously I suffered an acute inflammation on the right side of my lip. I had never had anything like that before, and it was very annoying, sometimes painful, and sometimes itchy.

"I went to a dermatologist who diagnosed it as herpes facialis. He described it as a development of vesicles on an inflammatory base. He gave me some ointment and told me it would probably start to dry up and heal over a period of the next several weeks.

"I was planning a trip abroad and I asked him, 'What is the longest you think it will take to heal?'

"He replied, 'Well, sometimes it can be pretty stubborn, and it could take six months or more to heal. I think it should be gone in three months at the outside.'

"As I said, I had been having some back pains at the

same time, so I went to see Dr. Reder for a treatment for my back. Dr. Reder inserted the applicators and I went into the lounge to relax. After about fifteen minutes, I had to go to the bathroom. While I was in there, I glanced into the mirror, and, to my amazement, most of the herpes inflammation had disappeared, leaving only a trace of redness.

"I rushed in to tell Dr. Reder about it, and he simply, said, 'That's one of the peripheral advantages. We don't charge for that. It comes with the main course.' "

The Man Who Lost His Erection

Gilbert George is about forty years old, quite handsome, and an excellent conversationalist. During my interview I learned very quickly that he enjoyed telling this story, and, although his tale involved some discussion of the intimate details of his love life, he was untroubled by it, and wanted to fill me in on everything.

Mr. George first married while he was still in his teens, and it took him a decade to decide that he and his wife were incompatible. He got a divorce when he was almost thirty, after which he fell in love with a newly hired secretary. By this time he was already in his early thirties, and his secretary was just twenty years old.

The marriage was a good one from many viewpoints. Gilbert had just shed one wife who was more of a competitor than a companion, and his new wife turned out to be an adoring, loving woman who thought that she had married the greatest man on earth. His new marriage was a happy one in many ways, but especially in their sex life. Gilbert's former wife had regarded sex as a chore that should be performed as infrequently as possible. The second Mrs. George, although no virgin, found Gilbert a satisfying lover, and she enjoyed sex with him. They took pleasure in each other, frequently reaching the heights of ecstasy.

When Gilbert fell into a pattern of sexual intercourse almost every morning and again almost every night, he decided to have a complete physical check-up just to reassure himself that his new regimen was appropriate for a man of his age. Gilbert and his wife had recently moved into a new apartment, and in the same apartment building a young doctor had offices. This made it unexpectedly convenient. Dr. Drummond gave Gilbert a thorough physical examination, including a stress test. Gilbert got a clean bill of health, except for one unpleasant surprise.

Dr. Drummond told him, "You're in excellent health, and everything checks out well, except that you have high blood pressure. I checked your pressure three times and it averages 150 systolic over 90 diastolic."

He continued, "Normal blood pressure for a man of your age should be less than 140, and when it goes above that, something needs to be done about it. The systolic pressure indicates the force of a contracting heart. Now take into account that your heart is beating about 72 times per minute. With your pressure, you have an enormous force pulsing through your body 72 times every minute. You can see that this is very bad for your overall health."

Gilbert George protested, "But, doc, I feel great. I haven't felt this good since I was a teenager. Is it possible there's a mistake? Maybe something is wrong with your instruments?"

Dr. Drummond shook his head. "The fact that you feel good is irrelevant because hypertension does not have any visible symptoms. People can walk around with high blood pressure for years, and not know it unless their pressure is checked by a doctor."

Gilbert asked, "Is it really important?"

The doctor replied, "Treating high blood pressure is

very important. What is happening to you is a 'pounding' pressure which is gradually damaging, or will damage, small arteries and other organs supplied with blood pumping from your heart. Unless you do something to reduce your pressure, it will ultimately affect your brain, your kidneys, and, of course, your heart itself. Your heart is beating against the higher pressure and working too hard. In effect, like a mechanical system that is being forced to work harder than it was designed to work, your heart will wear out earlier. You can suffer heart failure, kidney failure, and strokes."

Dr. Drummond gave Gilbert George a prescription for Lasix, and said, "I want you to come back in a week. These medicines affect different people in different ways and I want to prescribe the lowest possible dosage of the most effective medicine for you. That way we can reduce your blood pressure without unpleasant side effects. Once we work out the proper medication and the proper dosage, you won't have to see me so frequently."

Gilbert George had the prescription filled, and began to take the medicine according to the doctor's instructions. Once he overcame the initial shock of learning about his medical problem, he tended to forget about it, and to live in his usual style. However, a few days after he began to take Lasix, he made a very disturbing discovery. He could not achieve a satisfactory firm erection. No matter the stimulation, his penis remained flacid and uninterested in performing its duties.

Gilbert's head was still interested in sex, and he eagerly anticipated his morning and evening sexual activities with his nubile young wife. Unfortunately, in spite of his willing spirit, his flesh was weak. His penis refused to cooperate with his desires. It took a couple of days before he began to connect the loss of his erection with the hypertension medicine. When he did finally suspect the cause, he immediately discontinued the use of Lasix. A few days later, his erection returned as firm as ever.

A few days passed, and his performance continued to be as heroic as it ever had been. He decided to discuss it with friends, not telling them about the loss of erection, and simply try to learn if the treatment of hypertension was as important as Dr. Drummond had indicated. Those friends who knew something about the subject urged on him the importance of prompt and proper treatment for high blood pressure.

Reluctantly, he made another appointment with Dr. Drummond and diffidently told the doctor, "Doctor, the medicine you gave me had a very unfortunate side effect, so I stopped taking it. I couldn't get an erection, and let me tell you, I'm not at all happy about that."

Doctor Drummond smiled and replied, "Yes, I'm aware that that particular medication can possibly have such a side effect, and I'm sorry it did with you. I suppose I should have warned you about it. Well, don't worry. We'll try something else. You just keep reporting to me on the results. We'll try to find something that brings down your blood pressure, without bringing down anything else."

Dr. Drummond tried Aldactone, Catapres, Diuril, Esidrex, Hydradruril, Inderal, Salutensin, Reserpine, Aldomet, Ismeline, Apresoline, and Minipress. If the prescription worked on the hypertension, bringing the pressure down to normal parameters, then almost of a certainty Gilbert experienced loss of erection.

He shopped around for other doctors and other medicines. He even did some research on his own, attempting to arrive at an independent decision on the importance of controlling his pressure. By experimentation, he learned that if he discontinued all medication, within a few days his sex life had returned to normal. On the other hand, if he took a single dose of any one of the medicines, it immediately eliminated his ability to produce an erection. Unhappy with his need to make a choice, he nevertheless decided to discontinue all medication for hypertension. He opted to live with his high blood pressure, rather than sacrifice his sex life.

Gilbert George is a salesman, and he had to carry a heavy sample case. One day, while pulling his case out of his car, he felt a stab in his back. In his own words, "I think I twisted one of my vertebra by pulling on my sample case, and I felt a shooting pain down my right leg. I couldn't straighten up. My body was bent over, and when I tried to stand straight, I couldn't bear the excruciating pain down my right leg."

As soon as he could support his weight and bear the pain, Gilbert locked his car, took the first taxi he could get, and hobbled into Dr. Drummond's office, looking for relief.

The doctor said soothingly, "Fortunately, this condition you have is self-limiting. I would suggest that you get into bed and try to relax as much as you can for the next few days. I want you to take two aspirin every four hours and try to keep your mind on something else. Within a few days I'm sure you'll be okay."

Gilbert did as he was told, but, unfortunately, the doctor's prognosis was wrong. The pain persisted. After a week, he managed to drag himself off to work, but the pain continued to the point where it interfered with his daily routine. And, even more importantly to him, it made sexual intercourse painful, too. Any attempt to straighten his right leg brought on sharp shooting pains. It was the interference with his sex life, more than anything else, that pushed him into looking around for additional medical attention.

Dr. Drummond referred him to a rheumatologist, who was no help. He ran through the usual batting order of acupuncturists, chiropractors, and other healers of pain. Finally, in his rounds of medicine men, he heard of Dr. Milton Reder.

Dr. Reder's nasal therapy did not do much for his sciatic pain. He did get some relief, but by no means was it a cure. Some of the people he met in Reder's office told him that it was important to persist with the treatments, even to the extent of taking two a day, every day. One patient he spoke to told him, "I had almost the identical pain you have and I didn't get any relief until I started to take two treatments a day. Then after fifteen days the pain began to go away."

Although Gilbert wasn't happy over the prospect of such frequent treatments, he did start to visit Dr. Reder twice a day, and continued for two weeks. The pain lessened somewhat, but he wasn't really sure if it was going away just as a matter of elapsed time or if it was responding to the Reder therapy.

While he had been concentrating on controlling his high blood pressure, Gilbert George had purchased a home blood pressure kit. He had not taken his pressure for a considerable period of time because he was involved in the more immediate problem of relieving his sciatic pain. One night, while he was looking for something else, he came across the blood pressure kit. On the spur of the moment, he took his pressure. Much to his surprise, he discovered that his systolic pressure was 130. It hadn't been that low for a few years.

The next day, just to check himself, he went to see Dr. Drummond and told him about the low reading. Dr. Drummond took George's pressure and compared it with the previous readings on his chart. The doctor whistled and said, "Wow, I can hardly believe it! You must be doing something right. What have you been taking?"

Gilbert, still puzzled himself, replied, "I'm not taking anything."

Drummond asked, "Well, what are you doing? Or not doing?"

After a moment's thought, Gilbert said, "The only thing I can think of is those Dr. Reder treatments, which he calls sphenopalatine ganglion blockade. I've been getting them to try to get rid of the sciatic pain."

Dr. Drummond said, "I've heard about that, and about Dr. Reder, but I never heard that it worked for high blood pressure."

The next day when Gilbert returned to Dr. Reder's office, he asked: "Doctor, does this treatment do anything for high blood pressure?"

Reder replied, "Absolutely! It definitely lowers high blood pressure. Depending on the individual, it can sometimes have a reasonably lasting effect. In fact, it's one of the fastest ways I know to reduce high blood pressure. I use it on patients in an emergency when it becomes necessary to lower pressure in a hurry."

Today Gilbert George's sciatic pain is a distant memory. He no longer suffers from it, but he has learned to be supercareful when he moves his sample cases, to avoid causing any more damage to his back. He also checks his blood pressure three times a week. The moment it starts to edge up above 130, he visits Dr. Reder the next day.

He told me, "I need a treatment about once a week, and sometimes even twice a week. This keeps my pressure in check. And, what's more important to me, the nasal treatment has no effect on my sex life or on my ability to have an erection. I don't rely entirely on my own blood pressure readings, although I'm pretty good at it. Once a month I go to Dr. Drummond to have him check me. So far, the pressure stays down very well, and I don't have to take any of those hypertension medications."

CHAPTER XII

The Funny Side of the Business

Pain is a serious business, generally devoid of any humor. However, Milton Reder has a droll wit and is always ready for a joke. He manages to bring laughter to the suffering people assembled at 555 Park Avenue, in spite of their pain. Let me illustrate a typical Reder gambit which he uses from time to time to lighten the mood of his suffering patients.

One day unusual excitement filled the office because, in addition to ministering to the customary circus, Dr. Reder was training a young female physician in the technique of the sphenopalatine ganglion blockade. Dr. Blank was a practicing physician who had been working for some time in a Brooklyn pain clinic. She had heard of Dr. Reder and decided to add the SGB to her arsenal of pain-relief methods.

Dr. Reder does not normally examine patients with his stethoscope, but he did encourage Dr. Blank to do so. She had her stethoscope hanging around her neck in the timeless manner of all physicians, and she was checking out each patient who came into the treatment room.

One patient with breathing difficulties entered. Dr. Blank listened to the chest through her stethoscope and remarked, "Dr. Reder, the rales are quite evident. You can even hear the rhonchi."

She invited Dr. Reder to listen but he shrugged her off, muttering, "Clearly congested bronchial tubes. There's moisture in the air sacs."

Dr. Reder asked the young patient a number of questions and then remarked to Dr. Blank, "Our treatment has been fairly good for allergic asthma, and I think we ought to give it a try."

With this pronouncement, Dr. Reder dipped one of his four applicators in the cocaine mixture, squeezed them all together, and inserted one after the other into the nostrils of the waiting patient. The young man had been there before and he simply relaxed, waiting for the curative result of an application. Based on past performance, he had a reasonable expectation of relief.

After a few minutes, the patient rose and went into the outer room, where he sat down and picked up a magazine. Dr. Reder treated other patients, explaining to Dr. Blank what he was doing in each case. Half an hour later the young man came back into the treatment room to have the applicators removed.

Dr. Reder asked, "How do you feel?" The patient replied, "Much better, Doctor. I think this treatment did the trick."

The patient was ready to leave when Dr. Reder turned to Dr. Blank. "Why don't you listen through your stethoscope again? Let's see how we made out with the rales and rhonchi."

Dr. Blank inserted her stethoscope into her ears and

leaned forward to listen to the young man's chest. This unusual procedure attracted a number of patients as an audience.

Looking perplexed, Dr. Blank moved her stethoscope about on the patient's chest, listening intently. Finally she turned to Dr. Reder and said, "Doctor, the rales and ronchi have completely disappeared." Then, raising her voice, she continued, "You know, doctor, it's an absolute miracle!"

With a twinkle in his eye, Dr. Reder replied dryly, "Don't take it too seriously. This is no miracle. I just have these people come down from time to time from Central Casting. Most of them are just movie extras looking for a day's work, and I hire them to impress my patients." He then turned to the young man and said, "Okay, young man, you can pick up your money on the way out, and we'll call you when we need you again."

For a minute or two Dr. Blank looked puzzled. Her eyes made it clear that she was really debating the possibility that Dr. Reder's absurd remark was in fact the truth. Then she laughed and said, "Central Casting, my foot! You might be able to do it with quiet pain, but I heard those rales and rhonchi and no one is that good an actor! I'm sure that they were real, and the treatment eliminated them."

Dr. Reder laughed. "You would be surprised at the talented extras you can get from Central Casting."

Dr. Reder Walks on Water

A Reder patient of many years standing related the following story to me:

A physician brought in his mother, who had been suffering from chronic lower back pain. Her son had referred her to a variety of specialists, none of whom had been able to help her. Finally he himself put her on pain killers, but became afraid that she was becoming addicted to them. Finally, in desperation, he brought her to Dr. Reder.

Dr. Reder inserted the applicators and told her to relax. By the time it was necessary to remove the applicators, she was ecstatic over the relief from her nagging lumbo-sacral pain. Effusively, she made such remarks as, "Dr. Reder, what you do is magic. It's like a story from the Bible. You're like God, or at least one of his disciples. I believe you've been sent back to earth to do God's work."

Her son, the doctor, appeared annoyed at his mother's volubility. He said sharply, "Don't be absurd! This is a standard therapy procedure. Dr. Reder isn't Jesus, and he can't perform miracles."

Mother and son fell into an argument over whether Dr. Reder was in truth God's representative on earth, with neither participant willing to abandon his position. Finally, Dr. Reder, his voice revealing his amusement, intervened.

"Mom, you stick by your guns," Dr. Reder said to her. "You're right. In fact, I'll give you a demonstration."

He took a pitcher of water from his desk and carried it into the outer room. While everyone in the room watched with interest, he carefully poured a trail of water on the carpet. Then, with due solemnity, he walked firmly on the wet spots, saying to his patient, "See, Mom, I really can walk on water!"

The Balloon-Assisted Therapy

David Brenner, the famed comedian, and one of Dr. Reder's most devoted patients and admirers, told me this story:

One day a widely known New York orthopedic physician came to the Park Avenue office. Dr. Jones was both haughty and disparaging of the goings-on in the Reder ménage. He told anyone who would listen, "I don't believe that the sphenopalatine ganglion blockade will relieve sciatic or lumbo-sacral pain. Nevertheless, I've heard much about it, so I decided to investigate. You understand, I'm here to observe, but I might even try it on myself, just to further my investigation of the procedure."

Finally Dr. Jones introduced himself to Dr. Reder, saying, "I have some twinges of pain in my lower back, and I want to find out if your treatment could possibly help."

Dr. Jones's supercilious manner clearly conveyed his skeptical attitude toward the SGB. Everyone could see his total disbelief in the treatment. However, everyone there could also see that he was in some pain.

After Dr. Jones seated himself, Dr. Reder prepared and inserted the four applicators. Then he added an unusual touch. One of his patients had brought him some gas-filled balloons from Maxwell Plum's Restaurant. These were hanging from the ceiling in the waiting room. Now Reder walked into the waiting room, selected four of them, and carried them back to his office. He then attached the strings to the exposed tips of the applicators.

In a calm voice, he explained to Dr. Jones, "Some people have wider nostrils than others. You are one of those. In order to keep the applicators from slipping out, I use balloons to anchor them in place. I suggest you sit very quietly now, until it's time to remove them. That way they won't slip out of place and annoy you."

For half an hour the supercilious Dr. Jones sat very still, afraid to move any part of his body because of what might happen if he did. Meanwhile, aware of Dr. Reder's joke, patients kept coming to the door of the treatment room to peer in at the man with the balloons tied to his nose.

David Brenner remarks, "That was some sight! There sat this well-known, stiff-necked orthopod, sitting there with as much dignity as he could muster, with brightly colored balloons floating from his nose. Believe me, it wasn't easy for all of us to sit around with straight faces, acting as though this was the most normal procedure in the world."

The Rabbi Gives Thanks

A bearded rabbi, a long-time patient of Dr. Reder's, was awakened one morning by the sound of his wife quietly crying as she lay beside him in bed. During the night she had been stricken with a lower-back pain so severe she couldn't straighten out her legs. Every time she tried to stretch out in order to get out of bed, an intense pain knifed through her. Once it had been so acute that she thought she had lost consciousness for a short period of time.

The rabbi had been seeing Dr. Reder for many years for treatment of migraine headaches. He immediately decided that the best treatment for his wife would be the spheno-palatine ganglion blockade. He quickly dressed and summoned some friends to help him carry his wife to Dr. Reder's office.

With her legs still bent, two men picked up the rabbi's wife and placed her in a car. They lifted her out and carried her into the Reder office. She was still in her nightgown and robe, and unable to stretch out her legs.

Dr. Reder made her comfortable in a chair and inserted the applicators. As the blockade took effect, the rabbi's wife felt her pain diminish and ventured to straighten out her legs. After half an hour she could get up and walk around.

The rabbi was very excited over the quick relief for his wife, and fell to his knees in Reder's office, turning his face toward a window. He offered up prayers of thanksgiving to God for having blessed his wife with such a quick cure for her agony.

Dr. Reder watched him for a moment with some astonishment, and then, walking over to the kneeling rabbi, he said, "Rabbi, you're thanking the wrong one. It wasn't God who cured your wife. It was this cocaine." And he shook the bottle of cocaine solution under the rabbi's nose. Then he continued, "If you really feel like giving thanks, don't thank God, thank cocaine."

The Bent-Over Man Who Needed a Taxi

One day one of the patients in the office told me this story and swears to its authenticity.

He was approaching Dr. Reder's office one day and saw a man standing at the curb on Park Avenue, trying to hail a taxi. The man was bent over almost in a U-shape. His back paralleled the sidewalk, and he had turned his head sideways to watch for a cab. When he spotted one, he lifted his arm as best he could to try to hail it. The cab drivers, after one look at this apparition, just kept on going.

After watching for a few minutes, my informant walked over to him, tapped him on the shoulder, and said, "I have a car around the corner. I noticed you can't seem to stop a cab. Can I give you a lift?"

The man twisted his head around and peered upward, saying, "No, thanks, I'll be okay. Sooner or later I'll get a cab."

My informant tried to find out more about the bent-over man, finally saying, "You know, there's a doctor named Dr. Reder, whose office is on this very corner, who treats people with conditions like yours. I'm going in to see him now. I'll bet if you let him give you a treatment, you'll be able to stand straighter."

The bent-over man looked at his would-be benefactor and smiled. "I just *came* from there. You should have seen me before he started to treat me!"

Dr. Reder's Favorite Exercise

David Brenner, one of America's favorite comedians, also writes books of humor. His latest book is entitled, *Revenge Is the Best Exercise* (Arbor House, 1984). In it he turns exercise into a comical pursuit. The millions of people who enjoy David Brenner on stage and on TV will laugh their way through the pages of this book, and perhaps that in itself is a beneficial exercise. In one segment at the end he writes:

"I would like to take the time right here to tell you of one honest-to-goodness serious easy-to-do, totally beneficial exercise. The truth of the matter is that I have a chronic back problem, and I am limited in my ability to exercise.

"The following is an exercise that was suggested to me by one of my favorite human beings, Dr. Milton Reder of New York City. It works, honestly. It's fun, honestly. You'll love doing it, honestly. You'll feel like an idiot while you're doing it, honestly. The exercise consists of going into a body of water—a pool, lake or ocean—up to your chin and jogging for twenty minutes, taking a ten-minute break, and then going back in and jogging for another twenty minutes.

"The water keeps you buoyant and prevents you from straining any of your joints, such as ankles or knees, or damaging your internal organs, and the resistance of the water acts as a toning device. It's perfectly safe and will keep you in shape. The only precaution is to be sure that the water level never goes above your forehead. Once you get between one and six feet under water, jogging becomes more difficult, as does breathing. It is recommended you do not wear street clothes during the exercise. It is also suggested you do not do this exercise in the shipping lanes."

CHAPTER XIII

Highlights in the Life of the Miracle Worker

Dr. Milton Reder made it into the twentieth century by five days. He was born January 5, 1900, in Dayton, Ohio. He had two sisters, one of whom is a retired stockbroker, while the other was both an inventor and a lawyer until her death some years ago. Before he started school, his family moved to New York City. He attended city elementary and high schools and then continued his education at New York University.

After he earned his undergraduate degree, he enrolled in the medical school of New York University, which was then associated with Bellevue Hospital. The framed medical degree hanging on his office wall states he graduated from "New York University and Bellevue Hospital Medical College."

After receiving his degree in 1922, he was accepted by the Post-graduate Medical School (which later became the New York University Medical School), where he specialized in otolaryngology. He received his certification from the American Board of Otolaryngology in 1925. He became interested in the phenomenology of the sphenopalatine ganglion blockade during his medical residency.

In the practice of ear, nose and throat medicine, he had the opportunity to work with the ganglion in the treatment of cranial and facial pain. This work, together with his association with Dr. Sluder and Dr. Ruskin (his brother-in-law), led him in the direction of utilizing the anesthetization of the sphenopalatine ganglion to eliminate pain in other parts of the body.

After he received his certification in otolaryngology, he opened an office on Park Avenue, and got married. This marriage produced three children. The son of that marriage is an atomic physicist, one daughter works in television communications, and the other daughter works in transportation.

During World War II he held the rank of major in the Medical Corps, and was assigned to the European Theater of Operations. On D-Day he crossed the Channel to Omaha Beach, and moved on with the battles, working in field hospitals, where he performed emergency surgery.

He was discharged in 1946 with the rank of lieutenant colonel and once again opened an office on Park Avenue. He divorced his first wife and married Violet, with whom he had a son they named Milton A. Reder.

Young Milton is also a physician, and his proud father loves to brag about what an outstanding student his son was by the age of three. The family had to move into a specific neighborhood so that the child could attend what was considered to be one of the best public schools in the United States. Milton A. attended Johns Hopkins University and, after graduation, continued in Johns Hopkins Medical School, finally getting his certification in internal medicine in 1981.

Young Dr. Reder developed an interest in arthritis, and

began to use the sphenopalatine ganglion blockade experimentally in the treatment of that disease. As its value became apparent, he found himself using it on a regular basis. Today the younger man practices in Brookline, Massachusetts, where he specializes in both internal medicine and SGB treatments. When his father, for one reason or another, is unable to devote himself fully to his busy practice, Milton A. shuttles to New York to man the Park Avenue office.

A favorite story in the Reder family is how, when Milton A. was very young, he hated doctors because they stuck him with needles. As a result, no one told him that his father was a member of that frightening profession. Dr. Reder had a very busy practice, but made it a habit to take off Saturdays, when he went to the famed show biz hangout, the Friar's Club. In order to have some time with his son he would take the young boy with him.

At the Friar's Club Dr. Reder played cards with Goodman Ace, George Burns and other members of the theatrical profession. Watching his father playing cards with these men, the boy formed the impression that that was how his father earned his living. One day he discovered, to his great shock, that his father was a physician! It took some time for the boy to recover from this trauma.

The practice of medicine runs in the Reder family. The younger Doctor Reder is married to a physician. Their two year old son calls his father "Dr. Daddy," his mother "Dr. Mommie," and the older Dr. Reder is, of course, "Dr. Grandpa." In addition, Milton A.'s mother-in-law is an homeopath to the British Royal family and his wife's grandfather was Chief to the Royal College of Surgeons in Ireland.

After World War II Dr. Reder built up a Park Avenue practice in otolaryngology. He developed a good reputation among people in the entertainment industry. Performers had frequent need for his services because the very nature of their work frequently produced hoarseness or other vocal problems. Confronted with some of their complaints, he began to use the sphenopalatine ganglion blockade to relieve their problems.

When a performer obtained relief from pain and was enabled to go on with a performance, that person was likely to tell others about the success of the Reder treatment. As a result, many of his patients are actors and singers.

Dr. Reder is one of those fortunate people who have all the money they need to sustain them. When he first began to use the sphenopalatine ganglion blockade decades ago he charged $25 for each complete treatment. He has continued the treatment, and the charge for it, unchanged to this day.

Some years ago a grateful patient, one of the most astute investment counsellors in the country, who has requested he remain anonymous, put Dr. Reder into MCI stock at a price of $1 per unit. A few years later the counsellor sold out Dr. Reder's holdings in MCI with a substantial capital gain.

CHAPTER XIV

Some of Dr. Reder's More Famous Patients

More than one hundred of Dr. Reder's patients have been or presently are in *Who's Who in America*. They include members of Congress, Army generals, movie and TV superstars, singers, writers, artists, sculptors, and household names of diverse occupations and professions. When I started my interviews, some were reluctant to talk about their involvement with Dr. Reder.

Upon reflection, I realized that the superstar does not want his pain to become a matter of public record. Take, for example, Yul Brynner. His public image is of the perennial king, strong, stalwart, impervious. For obvious reasons, he doesn't want to distort that image with publicity about real physical problems.

Nevertheless, it is true that Yul Brynner was a Reder patient of long standing. Many of Dr. Reder's patients told me they had frequently observed him entering and leaving the office; his refrigerator still stands in the inner office as a testament to his presence. In spite of this evidence, he is reluctant to discuss the subject with anyone, maintaining his right to privacy in this area.

Dr. Reder, a strict observer of patient confidentiality, will not discuss anything concerning his patients. The information I have, I obtained from conversation with other patients, the media, and some private sources.

The Old Guard

Dr. Reder began offering the sphenopalatine ganglion blockade treatment in the late 1940's, after he returned from service in World War II. He was a natural choice as physician to the stars of the entertainment industry. His success with pain relief was balm for performers who had to make their appearances and conceal their pain no matter how much they suffered.

Many of them are now dead, but they were a voluble lot, and talked about Reder. Some of them even wrote about him. Tallulah Bankhead, in her autobiography, *Tallulah* refers to Dr. Reder (misspelling his name) with reverent awe. Because she used both tobacco and alcohol to excess, she suffered intermittant problems with her voice. When all else failed her, she called on Dr. Milton Reder for assistance.

Charles Revson, the founder of Revlon Cosmetics, was a regular. He learned very early about the pain relief afforded by the sphenopalatine ganglion blockade, and when, in later life, he contracted cancer, Dr. Reder visited him regularly in the hospital, bringing him relief from his severe pain.

Jose de Creeft, internationally known sculptor, was both a good friend and a regular patient. De Creeft is probably best known for his sixteen-foot-high sculpture of Alice in Wonderland, which stands in Central Park, New

York City, and for the statue titled "Poet" in Philadelphia's Fairmont Park. He died when he was almost one hundred years old, and Milton Reder's son delivered the eulogy at the funeral.

The David Brenner Story

David Brenner, the leading comedian of the new generation, is probably Dr. Reder's greatest booster today. At every opportunity he touts Dr. Reder and his pain-relieving treatments. He has talked about the treatment while doing a stint as guest host on the Johnny Carson show, on Regis Philbin's Cable Health News program, and on many other occasions.

When I asked for an interview, he told me the following story:

"I have been coming to Dr. Reder for more than ten years. I suffered from agonizing pain in my lower back which travelled into my arms and radiated down into my legs. I was on the road, giving frequent performances, and spending long hours on my feet. Everywhere I went I looked for any doctor who was recommended by anyone in the area.

"I visited chiropractors, orthopedic physicians, neurologists, and whoever else seemed to offer the possibility of any kind of relief.

"The one thing they all seemed to agree on was that I needed an operation. They said I had a herniated disc and double scoliosis of the upper and lower spine. I have degenerative spinal disease, both upper and lower. My L5 is herniated, I have bone spurs. My back is a mess!

"For more than six months I was in pain twenty-four hours a day. There I was, travelling all through the country giving performances, being humorous, making people laugh, and all the time I was suffering terrible pain.

"I had a cousin who died on the operating table while having a back operation. I also have a niece who had back surgery. She still has the pain, but now she also has a big scar on her back. One thing I knew for sure. No way was anyone going to put a knife in my back!

"One day I was talking to Sonny Buono, of Sonny and Cher fame, and he mentioned that he suffered from back spasms. He told me a story about one attack he had had, and a doctor who came to his hotel room and stuck wires up his nose. In half an hour he was okay and went on stage to give his performance.

"I thought a lot about what Sonny told me. I was worried about having someone shove wires up my nose, especially since I couldn't really tell if it would do any good. Well, anyway, it happened that I was in New York at the time, and I remembered my friend Steve had a bad back, too. So I told him about Sonny and his doctor. I urged Steve to see this Dr. Reder. Finally he did and got the treatment. Then I pushed him to tell me all about it. It didn't sound too bad, and Steve didn't appear to have suffered any ill effects from it. So next day I went.

"I'll never forget the first time I walked into that office. The place was really bizarre. Here were what appeared to be perfectly normal people sitting or standing around, doing perfectly normal things like reading or talking to each other, but all of them had these things sticking out of their noses. I didn't know whether to stare at them or pretend I didn't notice.

"Finally, it was my turn to see the doctor. He recognized me and went into his own comic routine. The first thing he said to me was, 'Did any doctor ever give you chicken soup to cure your back?'

"I answered, 'No, nobody ever gave me any chicken soup.'

"Then he wanted to know, 'Would you like to have some chicken soup?'

"'No, thanks,' I said dryly, 'I don't think it would help.'

"He didn't pay any attention to my answer. He opened a little refrigerator and took out a container of chicken soup and stuck it in front of me. I thought to myself, 'I'm getting out of this loony bin while I can. People are sitting around with things sticking out their noses, and the doctor is trying to coax me to eat cold chicken soup!' I started to turn around, then I thought, what the hell, I'm here already. I might as well stick around and see what else is going to happen.

"Finally he sat me down and put the applicators into my nose and told me to stay where I was. I sat there for twenty-five minutes, and then I got up and walked around. I couldn't believe it! Those wires had relieved my pain. For the first time in six and a half months I felt okay. I won't tell you I was all better, but at least half the pain was gone. I started to go for treatments every day and, after three weeks, I was one hundred percent better.

"Once I finished that first series of treatments, I was a believer. If I felt even a slight twinge in my back, I headed for Reder's office no matter how busy I was. Once I went without pain for two and a half years, and another time I was okay for four years. I didn't go that long without a treatment, of course, but I did go without the pain.

"One time I fell asleep on the plane flying to New York from the West Coast. When I woke up I couldn't get out of my seat. My body was frozen into a sitting position, and even the slightest movement gave me more pain than I could handle.

"They had to carry me off the plane and sit me in a cab. I went right to Dr. Reder's office, but this time it wasn't so easy because I couldn't stay around for a full course of treatments. I had contracts which took me on the road, and

I didn't get rid of the pain completely for seven months. But let me tell you, even so, Dr. Reder made it possible for me to keep on working.

"Now, whenever I'm in New York, which is where I live, incidentally, I come in for prophylactic treatments. I wish I had thought of starting that sooner. It would have saved me a lot of pain. Now I still get an occasional spasm, but as long as I keep up the treatments, it doesn't last long.

"I assure you, there's a big difference. Before, when I got a spasm, I'd just fall on the floor and lie there. Now when I get an attack, it hurts but I can still move slowly and get myself to Reder.

"I've seen all kinds of miracles in Dr. Reder's office. I remember one man whose head was all twisted and locked into a crazy position over his shoulder. I saw him get Reder's treatments, and in a short time he was cured.

"One day I got a phone call from a friend who had torn a ligament in his back in a tennis accident. He had been suffering for more than six months, and he complained to me that he didn't know what to do about it. I convinced him to see Dr. Reder. He did and he was cured. He's never had a problem with his back since then.

"I had another friend who was scheduled for surgery for a herniated disc. I convinced him to see Reder first, and he was cured without an operation.

"One of my friends suffered from vertigo. I sent him to Dr. Reder. After the first treatment, he felt better, and by the end of a week of treatment he was fine and didn't have to go back any more.

"When my son was born, his mother suffered a pinched nerve in her hip. Maybe six times a day she'd suddenly collapse from the pain. And normally she was quite an athlete. Her doctor told her it would take six months to a year for it to go away by itself. I didn't want her to wait.

"I brought her to Dr. Reder, and I still remember her

reaction. She took one look around the office, and decided the whole thing was absurd. She said she wouldn't even consider a treatment unless I took one first. Well, I didn't need one, but I took it anyway. When she saw that it was really quite simple, and didn't seem to bother me at all, she agreed to try one herself, but only under one condition. I had to pay her a hundred dollars—in advance. So I gave her the money, and she went on to take three more treatments. Then she was all better. Now I have to fight with her to get her to let me see my son. Believe me, I'm sorry I brought her here.

"A few years ago I overheard a man in the waiting room talking to someone. He complained of such pains in his back that he couldn't lift anything. His son was two years old and he had never been able to lift him. Incidentally, the man was from Paris, but from then on, every time he came to New York he visited Dr. Reder. He had to take only a few treatments to get rid of the pain, and for the first time he could pick up his son and carry him around.

"I can't resist using these incidents for practical jokes once in a while. One day the Frenchman was here taking a treatment and a woman sitting in the room heard his story. The man spoke English with a heavy French accent, but he was ready to tell everybody about his miracle.

"This woman was a new patient, and she had never had a treatment. She asked me, 'Is that story really true?'

"I replied, 'Absolutely! But you have to know there's one side effect. When that man first came here, he spoke perfect English. After he had a few treatments, he began to speak with that accent.'

"The woman looked at me suspiciously, then said, 'But I don't want an accent.'

"I shrugged my shoulders and looked sympathetic. She got up and began to move around the room, and then walked toward the door. I persuaded her to stay by convincing her that I was joking, and she didn't have to worry about getting an accent.

"Dr. Reder has treated a lot of famous people. He treated Rudolph Valentino, General George Patton, Randolph Churchill, John J. McCloy, John F. Kennedy, George C. Scott, Howard Hughes, George Burns, Phil Silvers and Hedy Lamarr. Goodman Ace was a patient and a good friend.

"Dr. Reder also treated Patricia Lawford, President Kennedy's sister. He's treated kings, including the King of Morocco. He even treated Alan King!

"When it looked like Whitey Ford, one of the great Yankee pitchers, wouldn't be able to pitch any more because of shoulder pains, Dr. Reder gave him three more years of pitching. In fact, a lot of athletes who thought they were all washed up came here for treatment and played again. I personally have sent him a number of performers, including Tom Jones, Mike Douglas, and Regis Philbin.

"Once, when I was doing the Carson show, I talked about Milton Reder and his work. Hundreds of people who heard me wrote to me asking about it. I couldn't answer everybody personally, so we made up a form letter. We told people that the treatment didn't work for everybody, but if they were interested, they could contact the doctor directly. I know for a fact that over a hundred people came to see him as a result of that one TV show.

"I've heard about a lot of interesting results. Once I went to an art show in Greenwich Village. I was looking at the paintings when a woman came up to me and said, 'Please wait here. My husband is dying to talk to you.' So I waited and in a few minutes this man comes over and he stares at me and his mouth drops open and he begins to cry.

"He finally said 'Mr. Brenner, I just have to thank you for saving my life.'

"He had been crippled by pain, and when he heard me

on TV, he went to see Dr. Reder. The treatments made him okay again.

"It's my opinion that the reason this treatment is not more widely accepted is because it's too cheap. If Dr. Reder charged $250 a visit, instead of $25, people would be standing on the sidewalk waiting to get in.

"It's like a friend of mine who had a used furniture business in a poor neighborhood. He had trouble selling anything. It was all junk anyway, the neighborhood was poor, and nobody bought any of it. I told him his trouble was, he was too cheap. He took my advice, put high prices on all his junk, advertised the stuff as antique, and guess what? He sold out!"

CHAPTER XV

Dr. Reder and the Press

One of the first times the press took notice of Dr. Reder was in an article in the April 9, 1965, issue of *Life* magazine. *Life* printed a large cartoon by E. R. Does, showing a man bending over while a group of people worked on his spine. The story that accompanies the cartoon is about Toots Shor, the well-known New York restaurateur.

Shor tells the story about one time when he was in an airplane on his way to St. Louis to attend a wedding. He went over to talk to Grace Kelly, who was also on the flight. While sitting on the arm of a seat, he had a back seizure. He made it to the wedding, but he insists that the only thing that got him through it was the booze. He said "I anesthetized myself."

When he got home, he limped for weeks from one doctor to another. Someone told him to go see the doctor who "sticks wires up your nose." He replied, "You must be kidding. I've got a bum back." His informant insisted that the doctor really could cure bad backs with wires in the nose.

Shor, although skeptical, finally did visit Dr. Reder. He sat through the treatment, feeling foolish, but waiting patiently to see what would happen. At last Dr. Reder said, "Now bend over and tie your shoes."

Toots Shor says, "I did. I'm telling you it's the Lourdes of Park Avenue. You've got to see this place."

The author of the article visited Dr. Reder's office to observe the treatments for himself and to speak to the patients. The story is, in brief, similar to that found on the pages of this book. It is an upbeat, favorable impression.

At the other end of the scale is a pejorative article in *New York* magazine, which belittles the treatment and emphasizes without foundation that it leads to cocaine addiction. The article is poorly researched, as, for example, in the description of the use of "five" wires placed in the nose. The maximum ever used is four. At times the treating physician will use only two applicators if the nostrils are small or the patient has a deviated septum, but five applicators are never used. The article is filled with similar inaccuracies.

More recently (May 6, 1985) the *New York Post* gave some publicity to a legal action involving a New Jersey housewife. In actual fact, investigation of the case discloses that the patient in question was treated by Dr. Janet Jacub, a psychiatrist, who used office space on the same floor as Dr. Reder's office at 555 Park Avenue, in the late '70s. Dr. Jacub was in no way associated with Dr. Reder, and the patient in question saw Dr. Jacub, not Dr. Reder.

As a result of the publicity the *New York Post* gave the case, many celebrities protested to the paper, pointing out that Dr. Reder had cured them of pain. Designer Jacques Bellini called the *Post* to report, "I was in traction two months. They wanted to operate on me. I couldn't walk. I was crawling. I had tried everything." Bellini said that he had friends carry him to Dr. Reder's office where, within twenty minutes of the start of treatment, his pain was gone and he could walk again. He concluded, "He saved my life!"

Lew Rudin, President of the Association for a Better New York, reported to the *Post* that he went to Dr. Reder for treatment of a bad back. He said, "He did such a good job on me I haven't had to go back except to say 'hello.' He's a wonderful, a good, old friend of mine."

Marvin Mitchelson, the well-known California divorce attorney who invented palimony, reported to the *Post*, "He's a marvelous physician. He helped me immeasurably with my chronic neck pains." (In my interview with Mitchelson, he told me that he regularly flew to New York just to take a treatment whenever he felt twinges in his back. In addition, if he is on the East Coast on business, he always stops in to see Dr. Reder and to take a treatment.)

From time to time there are little flurries in the press about Dr. Milton Reder and his treatment. Dr. Reder takes it all very equably, regarding the comments, whether good or bad, as of little significance. In discussing the article in *New York* magazine, his comment to me was, "What they say in a magazine like that is not very important. What is important is to relieve the pain of the patients who come in here looking for help."

CHAPTER XVI

In Which I Discuss What I Have Learned About Pain

It would require an individual with an inverted bump of intellectual curiosity to have done the research for this book without acquiring a deep interest in the subject of pain. Even the langauge of pain is intriguing. No one talks about pain without using at least one descriptive adjective. The range runs from unbearable, horrible, terrible, and similar descriptive terms to exquisite, burning, shooting, and the like. Pain has developed a complete vocabulary of its own.

What Is Pain?

After much deliberation, I conclude that pain, like many other concepts—such as time, love, and beauty, and even broader terminology like pornography—is easily understandable, but impossible of definition. Paraphrasing the famed words of Supreme Court Justice Stewart, we all know pain when we feel it, but it is impossible to describe.

In order to arrive at a more precise concept, let's consult some authorities on the subject. We begin with Mr. Webster's Unabridged Dictionary. That authority's Second Edition offers a series of definitions for the word "pain." They are as follows:

"1. Punishment; suffering or evil inflicted as a punishment for crime or connected with the commission of a crime; penalty; fine.

"2. A form of consciousness characterized by desire of escape or avoidance and varying from slight uneasiness to extreme distress or torture. An affliction or a feeling proceeding from derangement of functions, disease or bodily injury, 'the pain of Jesus Christ.'

"3. Distressing uneasiness of mind: mental suffering; grief.

"4. The throes or travail of childbirth; labor.

"5. The torment of hell or purgatories; hell; purgatory.

"6. Chiefly cruel. Labor; toilsome effort; care or trouble; as, to be at pains, or take pains, to learn the facts; here is a reward for your pains.

"7. Psychol. A sensation varying in quality from prick to ache, commonly aroused by a stimulus that injures or nearly injures the skin or tissues, usually but not always unpleasant, and leading to avoiding reactions."

I question very much whether a being from another planet where pain has been eliminated, landing on earth and reading those definitions, could possibly understand what constitutes pain. Having read through them a few times, I believe it is like trying to define water by saying, "Water is what makes you wet when it rains."

Pain as an attribute of life has an importance that ranks just below hunger, thirst and sex. Dr. Steven F. Brena, in his book, *Chronic Pain: America's Hidden Epidemic*, introduces his subject with the following comment:

"Pain is one of the most important concerns of humankind and a factor that has influenced history. This is documented in the records of every race and civilization: in the cave drawings of prehistoric man, in the oldest written documents of ancient China, on Babylonian clay tablets and papyri written in the days of the Pyramid builders, on Persian leather documents, and on the parchment scrolls from Troy."

That great wordsmith, John Milton, in *Paradise Lost*, described pain as "perfect miserie."

What the Doctors Can Do About It

Unfortunately, pain, like the common cold, has evaded the most arduous research efforts of the medical profession. Medical men have learned to use the laser as a replacement for the surgical scalpel, and the computerized scan to image the innermost secret of the human body. The modern world enjoys medical marvels without number. Unfortunately for the sufferer, simple pain still escapes the ministrations of the physician.

Drs. Smoler and Schulman, in a recent book titled *Pain Control: the Bethesda Program*, say in their introduction: "The medical miracles we constantly hear about increase our confidence in doctor's know-how to fix us when we break. Though we accept that the doctors are still working on major breakdowns like cancer, we assume that they have no trouble with everyday repairs like a strained back or an inflamed joint.

"No one has to tell you how this fairy tale is totally shattered when pain strikes. Some of you find that medicine does not have the answer to everything, and that the answers you do get are not even the same from doctor to doctor. You are trapped in a cave, screaming to get out, but no one hears you."

Why Pain Is So Elusive

The human body is as complex an organism as the mind of man can possibly conceive. We frequently think of modern main frame computers as being inordinately complex. As one computer specialist commented, after studying medicine and biology in preparation for writing a computer program, "If all the computers in the world were put together into a single giant computer, they would not be one millionth as complex as the human body."

The Dermatomes

When a human spermatozoon fertilizes a human ovum, a human embryo is formed. Although the embryo is microscopic, it consists of thirty-two basic segments. Each one is called a dermatome and each dermatome will eventually become an area of the human body. However, the dermatomes, for reasons known only to God, are not confined to an area which is logical to our current view of the body. For example, let us examine one dermatome (sometimes referred to as C8) in the neck. This will include one spinal neck vertebra and all the surrounding ligaments and nerves, and will travel down along the lower portion of the forearm, cover half the palm of the hand and three fingers—the little finger, the ring finger and the middle finger.

This knowledge is very important in the understanding of pain because pain tends to travel within its own dermatome. For example, imagine sustaining an injury to the base of the neck. You may have pain at the point of impact, or you may not. You may, in fact, feel pain only down the back of your arm. This is because the back of the neck, the upper arm, and the forearm are part of the same dermatome.

The dermatome story gets even weirder when we consider the pain that occurs when a disc in the lower part of the back presses on the nerve, or similarly when a lower back ligament is strained. With either of these types of injury there is a good possibility that you will feel pain down the outer part of the leg, across the foot and running into the big toe. You will not necessarily feel any pain at all in the lower back where the injury really is. In short, if you injured any part of the body, you can feel the pain in any part of the injured dermatome.

It would then be logical to expect that physicians who specialize in pain relief would map out the pain areas and end up with an understanding of how to apply the location of a pain to the cause of the pain. However, Mother Nature planted a joker at this point. The dermatomes are not precisely the same in every human being. They can actually cover different areas, different places and different sizes in different people.

The fact that the human body is made up of dermatomes creates another interesting problem: There is actually very little real perception of pain in the internal parts of the body, but any internal cause of pain is referred to the surface. For example, conditions generating pain in the heart follow a path to the center of the chest, the left shoulder and along the thin strip extending down the inner side of the left arm into the little finger.

Referred Pain

The existence of the dermatomes is one of the reasons why we have injuries at one point of the body and feel the pain in another. On the other hand, other instances of referred pain cannot in truth be blamed on dermatomes.

Dr. Gerald M. Aronoff, Director of the Spaulding Pain Center in Boston, points out that the man who is having a heart attack and feels the pain down his arm is not displaying the only example of referred pain. He says neck pain presents a similar situation. "People may feel pain in their hands. We have patients who say they need treatment for wrist pain, when the real problem is in the neck."

The dental literature is replete with instances of individuals who complain of pain in the teeth, even to the extreme of having them removed, only to learn eventually that the teeth were okay and the pain came from a different nerve in the head.

Dr. Hubart Rosenoff, of the Comprehensive Pain Center at the University of Miami, one of the major pain-treatment and pain-research centers in the world, says that, although a patient may have a diseased hip, the pain can be felt in the inside of the knee. He also cites incidents where individuals suffering from severe abdominal problems experience pain in their shoulders.

Trigger Points

At the present time the complete compendium of referred pain is baffling to physicians. Of course, they know the more common paths that pain follows, such as the pain of an injured back, which travels along the sciatic nerve into the leg, causing leg pain. This is so common that they have thoroughly mapped it out.

However, other pains which are essentially referred pains are not so well documented medically. Medical researchers are learning about areas called "trigger points." In feeling along the skin and palpating the muscles of patients in pain, certain tender spots have been encountered.

When the examiner presses these spots, the patient reports pain at some other site of the body. These trigger points are beginning to be mapped out, and seem to offer a good source of information which may lead to discovery of the location of the pain.

More recently, doctors have discovered how to inject local anesthetics—as, for example, novocaine—into a trigger point. Sometimes temporarily, and sometimes permanently, the injection relieves a pain existing in some other part of the body.

Dr. Janet G. Travell is a leading expert on trigger points and referred pain. Dr. Travell, now 85, still practices medicine in Washington, D.C.

During the Depression of the thirties and on into the early forties, Dr. Travell worked with patients in a New York City hospital, specializing in arm and shoulder pain. As so often happens, she became interested in the subject because she herself suffered from shoulder pain. Using herself as a patient, she discovered that she could produce the shoulder pain by pressing a spot near the shoulder blade. She researched the medical literature and discovered descriptions of similar findings.

Following some of the procedures outlined, she began to test her patients. She learned that heart patients would experience the typical heart-related pain when she poked them in the shoulder blades. She began to treat these patients with novocaine injections at the trigger point, and was able to relieve their pain.

Primarily as a result of this work, she became the attending physician to Senator John F. Kennedy, and in 1961 received the appointment as White House physician when Kennedy became president.

For those interested in pursuing the subject further, much of this information can be found in a 1983 publication which Dr. Travell wrote with Dr. David D. Simmons. The book is entitled *Myofacial Pain and Dysfunction, the Trigger Point Manual* (published by Williams & Wilkins).

The Paths of Pain

Located throughout the body are sensors. These sensors are receptors of sensation, particularly sensations such as heat, cold and pain. The sensors are concentrated in certain parts of the body—for example, the fingers and the hands. They are few and far between in other areas—for example, within the body in the abdomen, and on the surface of the body in the back, on the buttocks and between the shoulders.

At one time there was a fraternity rite in which the candidates for initiation were shown hot coals and told they would be branded on the back with the fraternity symbol. The candidate would see one of his tormentors pick up a hot coal with a pair of tongs. Then he would feel what he assumed was the hot coal pressed against his back.

In actual fact, an ice cube was substituted, out of sight of the candidate. Because the sensors are few and far between in the middle of the back, the body cannot quickly identify the true sensation. Therefore, the brain, interpretor of all sensation, having been preconditioned to expect burning pain, signalled the expected burning. It did, indeed, feel to the harried candidate for initiation that he had been branded by a hot coal.

From the sensor, the recipient of the stimulus, the sensation travels along a nerve or nerves into the spinal cord. The spinal cord is the mainstream for the transmission of sensation, and it receives a constant barrage of input, conveying a diversity of sensation, including pain, to the brain. The brain advises its host of the meaning of the signals it receives. When it receives the signal called "pain," the brain passes on the information that pain is being experienced, and includes the location from which the pain emanates.

The brain is able to mediate the pain, deciding whether to continue the sensation, or put it on hold. Many reports have been documented of soldiers who had received acutely painful wounds, and reported no pain until they arrived at the MASH unit or at the field hospital. The obvious implication of this is that, in the heat of battle, the brain decided it was the wrong time to communicate pain. Therefore, the sensation of pain was "turned off" until a more favorable moment.

Important to the distribution of pain signals is a portion of the brain called the thalamus. This is sometimes described as a central relay station. The thalamus plays a significant role in handling, interpreting, and conveying pain signals. Multiple inner connections exist from the thalamus to higher brain centers, such as the cerebral cortex, where finer interpretations and discriminations as to pain take place, and judgments are made.

Acute and Chronic Pain

We can now arrive at an understanding of a major difference between two types of pain. When you touch a hot stove and your fingers hurt unbearably, nature provides an emergency pathway in which the electro-chemical impulse that runs from the burned finger to the interpretation section of the brain takes priority over all other signals, and travels at lightning speed up the neural pathways to be interpreted.

The speed is almost instantaneous, so that you pull your fingers away from the hot stove seemingly at once. In effect, the major function of acute pain is to advise the body that something undesirable is happening, and should be corrected immediately. It is the same kind of pain reaction that occurs when a portion of the body is cut or severely bruised, or a ligament is strained or a tendon pulled. These pains are acute, severe, instantaneous and vital to the preservation of the integrity of the body for future use. Acute pain has a significant purpose in the preservation of human life.

Chronic pain, on the other hand, is a different story. It is probable that some day we will understand the meaning and purpose of chronic pain, at least as well as we understand acute pain.

At the present time we can discern little meaning and no purpose. For example, many people suffer from chronic headaches of one kind of another. Once a brain tumor is ruled out, there appears to be little reason for the chronic pain of a headache. Yet, the headaches come and go throughout the life of the patient, impairing the quality of life, and making existence a hell.

The spine is, of course, the major source of chronic pain. Anthropologists say that man was never meant to stand upright, and that if man traveled on all fours, he would not have backaches. Whatever the truth of their belief, it is of no comfort to the man with a backache.

The Memory of Pain

Experts on chronic pain say that the body has built-in "forgetters" which help to erase the memory of acute pains. One major example of this phenomenon, according to reports by women, is that they cannot really remember the true sensations of labor or delivery. This may be Nature's way of insuring that women will be willing to become pregnant after once having experienced labor and child birth.

On the flip side, the memory of chronic pain is vividly retained. People can describe in vivid detail, limited only by individual vocabulary, the chronic pain they experience.

Superficially, this sounds like an excellent arrangement on the part of Nature, since the body can use acute pain for the purpose of discontinuing some act which produces a harmful effect on it (touching a hot stove or impaling a limb on a nail), without leaving behind a traumatic memory.

The remembrance of chronic pain makes it possible to take corrective action against deep-rooted injury or disease. This arrangement may sound okay on the surface, but if you think about it further, you begin to see the flaws. The brain, which contains the memory of pain, has a memory bank which appears to be too efficient. For example, an amputee will frequently feel pain in the missing limb, a condition sometimes called "phantom limb pain." Unfortunately for the victim, it is as intense as any other pain.

As a result of a sciatic nerve injury some years ago, the area surrounding my right big toe is numb. When the neurologist pricks the toe with a pin, I feel no sensation. However, I regularly feel severe pain in that toe just as though I had just stubbed it. Why? And who needs it?

Anesthesiologists report that they can use nerve blocks for temporary elimination of pain impulses along certain neural pathways both in peripheral nerves and in the spinal cord. The block controls pain and provides analgesia to permit surgical procedures which would otherwise be extremely painful. On the other hand, when certain chronic-pain patients receive nerve blocks that produce total numbness, they report the pain persists in the area which has been theoretically rendered completely insensitive.

There is another example of that pain-sensation area of the brain which seems to inflict itself on man for no apparent reason. Spinal stenosis is a narrowing of the spine, causing pressure on those spinal nerves which travel down into the legs. The pressure produces pain in either one or both legs.

Research indicates that if the spinal stenosis is diagnosed early enough and surgical intervention takes place immediately to eliminate the pressure on the nerve, the patient is frequently rendered pain-free thereafter. However, if the spinal stenosis persists over a long period of time, the body acquires total memory of the pain. After this, if surgical intervention takes place, and the pressure on the nerve is eliminated, theoretically the patient should be pain-free. Unfortunately, the memory of pain persists, and many patients report that the pain down the leg or legs continues, notwithstanding successful surgery.

No one really understands why the brain memorizes chronic pain and persists in recalling it after the real pain is gone. Nevertheless, the phenomenon does exist and must be taken into account in any attempt to understand pain. I have reviewed the current theories concerning pain primarily to point out that the fact that the SPG blockade eliminates pain for many people is no more mysterious than a hundred other imcomprehensible aspects of pain.

Someday scientific researchers will discover the reason why, and even discover how to eliminate the pain recall. At the moment, and into the foreseeable future, memorization does exist for reasons unknown.

Pain and the Experts

An increasing number of medical doctors are beginning to recognize the significance of pain. Currently, the International Association for the Study of Pain sponsors an annual World Congress. In 1984 they held their meeting in Seattle, Washington. Some of the experts in the field of pain relief have even coined a new name for the specialty: analgesiology.

While gathering the material for this book, I wrote to many of these experts and a number of them took the time to reply. A typical letter came from Professor P. W. Wall, D.M., F.R.C.P., Director of the Cerebral Functions Group of the Department of Anatomy and Embryology at University College, London, England. Dr. Wall replied, in full:

Dear Mr. Gerber,

I'm aware of the claims that have been made for the effectiveness of a block of the sphenopalatine ganglion. I'm not aware of any clinical trial of this method which has been conducted with the following standard criteria.

1) Certified diagnosis.
2) Random allocation into two groups.
3) Double-blind treatment with local anesthetic or placebo.
4) Assessment of effect by an observer who did not know if the patient was in the treatment or placebo groups.

I believe a trial of this nature is essential before results of therapeutic effect are accepted.

Sincerely,
Professor P. D. Wall

Unfortunately, that is the typical attitude of a large percentage of the members of the medical profession.

On a more hopeful note, a scientific study is currently under way in Boston and its results should be known in the near future. In the interim thousands of people all over the world are benefiting from treatment by doctors who are willing to experiment with a pain-relieving procedure, even though it has not yet been scientifically proven in the laboratory by the double-blind test.

While doing research in the field of pain, I encountered

an analogous situation. In 1964 Norman Cousins, one of America's literary giants, suffered a crippling and painful disease.

He contracted a collagen illness which attacks the connective tissue. This falls into the category of rheumatic and arthritic disease. Collagen is the fibre-like substance which binds cells together. As Cousins says in his book, *Anatomy of an Illness* (New York: W. W. Norton Co., 1979), "In a sense, then, I was becoming unstuck.

"Experts from a New York clinic were called in and confirmed the diagnosis and added that it appeared to be 'ankylosing spondylitis' which in effect meant that the connective tissues in the spine were disintegrating."

His physician gave him one chance in 500 to recover, and the specialists stated flatly that they had never personally witnessed a recovery from this condition.

Norman Cousins, former editor of *Saturday Review*, author of several books, literary representative of the United States throughout the world, is a resourceful, inventive and pugnacious individual. The more he thought about it, the more convinced he became that this was not a problem to leave solely in the hands of the medical pundits. He knew that to get better he'd have to do it himself.

Cousins put his *Saturday Review* research assistants to work looking up medical points pertinent to his condition. It gradually became clear that he would not get better if he continued to take the prescribed drugs ordered by the medical "experts," drugs ranging from phenylbutazone to aspirin.

He concluded that his body would not have a chance of mending the damage to it if it were inhibited from recovery by numbing pain killers. However, he believed that if he stopped taking the drugs, he would not be able to handle the pain.

Making his personal analysis of pain, he determined that

an antidote or analgesic could well be obtained from laughter. Thereupon, he left the hospital and took up residence in a hotel, where he began a regimen designed to produce laughter. Alan Funt of "Candid Camera" sent some of his classic TV shows, and Cousins added some old Marx Brothers films from his home film library.

He made the joyous and somewhat startling discovery that ten minutes of "genuine belly laughter had an anesthetic effect which would give me at least two hours of pain-free sleep." When the analgesic effect wore off he would switch to some other form of humor which frequently also would lead to a pain-free period. He experimented with a variety of laughter-producing material. He had his nurse read him jokes and excerpts from classic humor.

Utilizing a combination of laughter and vitamin C therapy, and completely eliminating sleeping pills and other drugs, he began to recover. At first he was miraculously able to move his thumb without pain. Months later, he could raise his arms enough to remove a book from a shelf.

In spite of the pessimistic prognosis of the orthodox medicine men, Cousins recovered sufficiently to return to full-time work at the *Saturday Review*. He still felt some pain, but it no longer prevented him from playing tennis and golf, and enjoying time at the piano keyboard.

When Norman Cousins began to write about his personal experiences in dealing with a debilitating disease, and relieving himself of the attendant pain, the "experts" scoffed. As could well be anticipated, no physician adopted laughter as a potential pain-killer. Unfortunately, from the viewpoint of the patient who might have used such therapy, no scientific double-blind study supported the claim.

Recently, however, Dr. William Fry of Stanford University School of Medicine began to do some serious research on the value of laughter in medicine. He reports that laughter increases respiratory activity, oxygen exchange, muscular activity, and the heart rate. It also serves to stimulate the cardiovascular system, the sympathetic nervous system, the pituitary gland, and the production of the hormones called catecholamines. The latter stimulate the brain to produce endorphins, natural pain-reducing enzymes with a chemical composition not unlike that of morphine and heroin. Some of Dr. Fry's conclusions are described in the June, 1985, *Newsletter* of the University of California at Berkeley.

Experimentation in the field is ongoing. The University of California at Santa Barbara is working on a laughter project, investigating the effect of laughter on the human body. In one experiment, the group recently reported that laughter reduced stress just as well as the more complex bio-feedback program does.

To date no one has yet undertaken a double-blind study to prove that laughter can control pain. It is amusing to speculate on how a protocol could be designed for implementing such a study, or just what could be used as a placebo. In any event, until such a study is made, Norman Cousins to the contrary notwithstanding, I assume that those who agree with Professor Wall's position will not accept laughter as a therapy. To paraphrase David Brenner, "The doctors won't accept it because laughter is too cheap."

CHAPTER XVII

Is the SGB Treatment a Placebo?

While doing the research for this book, in addition to checking general and medical libraries in several states, I wrote letters of inquiry to world-famous experts in the field of pain. Some of them reported they knew nothing about the sphenopalatine ganglion blockade. Others wrote me, in effect, that in their opinion any benefit the patient received from the SGB was a "placebo effect."

In order to develop a completely rounded picture, I had to investigate the placebo effect. The word "placebo" is the future tense of the Latin verb *placere*, meaning "to please," and "placebo" means, "I shall please . . . " In short, it is a medicine given to the patient for the purpose of pleasing rather than curing.

A standard medical dictionary definition is that a placebo is a medicine which has no drug effect. It is given to humor the patient, and perhaps to allow the physician to charge for its psychological effect. The placebo also has its place in medical research, where it is used as a control.

Is the SGB Treatment a Placebo?

Unquestionably, a placebo has a definite effect on pain in a certain percentage of patients. Drs. Smoller and Schulman, in their book *Pain Control,* report that "Under certain circumstances, placebos have alleviated pain, healed ulcers, corrected abnormalities, relieved hay fever, stopped coughs, and lowered blood pressure. It is pretty amazing to realize that a pill with nothing in it can do all of this, and more."

Recently experimenters have begun to comprehend the biochemical aspects of a placebo. It has been recognized for a long time that the placebo has a psychological effect in that the patient anticipates that the pain will be relieved, or the condition improved, and the mind turns the anticipation into a certainty. Even a beginning student in psychology can understand this phenomenon.

I have observed what happens to Dr. Reder's patients, and as a result I incline strongly to believe that this particular placebo effect does *not* apply to them.

In the first place, the placebo effect, from a psychological viewpoint, is based upon the patients's anticipation of a particular result from the medication. The patient is predisposed to expect relief or cure from the treatment, so, in essence, the result is predetermined in the patient's mind.

Among Dr. Reder's patients I have yet to meet a single one who contemplated in advance that the insertion of applicators into the nose could, or would, relieve the particular condition which had produced the pain. On the contrary, I have heard, over and over, the same comment from the hundreds of patients I interviewed: "I was sure those wires in my nose wouldn't help at all." Later almost every patient who experienced relief of pain from the treatment admitted surprise and even bewilderment over the beneficial results.

The usual comment is, "I haven't the slightest idea how

this works, or why it did me any good. What I do know is that it did relieve my pain."

Under normal circumstance, this would end that part of the story. At this point I feel it incumbent upon me to report that recent experiments suggest that the placebo effect is something more than a psychological reaction. It appears that certain stimuli, including the placebo, can cause the brain to manufacture its own remarkable pain killers. These are sometimes referred to as endorphins.

Some recent experiments shed new light on the placebo. For example, patients who are familiar with the effects of morphine and know its benefits as a pain reliever were told they would receive morphine. Instead, a sugar pill was administered to some, together with a dose of naloxone. The latter drug, in proper dosage, completely neutralizes morphine's effect. Patients who received the sugar pill and would normally be expected to show some placebo effect as a result, as evidenced by other experiments with the same patient, showed no effect after being given the naloxone.

This experiment clearly indicates the presence of a substance in the body which simulates the effect of morphine, and it is the production of that substance which produces pain relief after a placebo is administered. Naloxone, which neutralizes morphine, apparently also neutralizes whatever chemical the brain produces in the manufacture of its own pain killers, the endorphins.

A recent experiment conducted by Jon D. Levine and Newton C. Gordon, of the University of California at San Francisco, indicates that placebos work totally outside the context of psychological effects. These researchers administered either a placebo, or morphine, or naloxone to 96 dental patients receiving dental surgery, at the time when the dental surgical anesthesia was wearing off. The patients received either open, hidden, or machine-regulated doses of the various substances mentioned above. Many of the patients had no idea of when the dose would be administered.

The results were startling. Pain increased in all cases when naloxone was administered. This would be expected because, as we've already seen, naloxone neutralizes opiate effect. But both morphine and the placebo reduced pain about the same amount, even though in both cases the patient had no knowledge of which drug was administered, if any. In fact, the patient was generally uninformed as to whether any drug at all would be given.

The experimenters concluded that the brain manufactures natural opiates, stimulated by the administration of almost any substance. If the placebo effect is produced by inducing the brain to manufacture natural opiates to kill pain, it then becomes completely understandable why the sphenopalatine ganglion blockade might work. The treatment is administered to a spot in the head very close to the brain. It may well be that the treatment stimulates the brain to manufacture endorphins to relieve the pain wracking the body, regardless of its location.

Appendices

APPENDIX I

Physicians Who Offer the SGB

The following is not a complete list of every practitioner who offers the SGB. Some physicians who perform the treatment have requested that they not be included in this listing. Each has personal reasons for the request and I have respected them, with one exception, which will appear below. With that one exception, all names listed here appear with permission.

MARC FREEDMAN, M.D.

Dr. Freedman has offices at 13908 Lakeshore Boulevard, Suite 250, Hudson, FL 33567. His telephone number is (813) 863-1591. Dr. Freedman was trained by Dr. Richard S. Klein (listed hereafter). He is Board Certified in Internal Medicine.

SEYMOUR M. GLUCK, M.D., F.A.C.P.

Dr. Gluck is Board Certified in Internal Medicine, and practices at 1204 Beach 9th Street, Far Rockaway, NY 11691. His telephone number is (718) 327-8585. Dr. Gluck frequently appears in Dr. Reder's office on Park Avenue and serves as an excellent substitute for Dr. Reder when Dr. Reder is sick or for some other reason cannot attend his patients.

SAMUEL GOLDFARB, M.D.

Dr. Samuel Goldfarb has his office at 19 West Central Avenue, Onset, MA 02558. His telephone number is (617) 295-0326. Dr. Goldfarb studied under Dr. Richard S. Klein (listed hereafter) and has performed the SGB hundreds of times. He was an anesthesiologist at the local hospital for many years, but has now given up that portion of his practice.

PAUL GUSMORINO, M.D.

Dr. Gusmorino was trained by Dr. Reder. He maintains his office at 301 E. 17th Street, New York, N.Y. 10003, and his phone number is (212) 734-3927. Dr. Gusmorino specializes in multi-disciplinary therapy for chronic pain. He is also associated with the Hospital for Joint Diseases Orthopedic Institute in New York City.

RICHARD S. KLEIN, M.D.

Dr. Klein practices in the Commerce Building, 1940 Commerce Street, Yorktown Heights, NY 10598. His telephone number is (914) 962-5577. Dr. Klein, who studied under Dr. Reder, has in turn trained several physicians. He has also written extensively on the SGB. He presented an abstract entitled "World Congress on Scientific Acupuncture, Sphenopalatine Ganglion Block in Chronic Pain." This was presented in Vienna, Austria, in October, 1983. He also presented a similar abstract at the 1983 meeting of the Canadian Pain Society. We have earlier written about the report which he presented at the International Congress on Pain in Seattle in 1984 (see Appendix III). Dr. Klein is one of the leading experts in the field.

N. J. MINTZ, D.O.

Dr. Mintz practices at 75 Bloomfield Avenue, Denville, NJ 07834. He studied under Dr. Reder and has performed the SGB for several years.

MILTON A. REDER, M.D.

Dr. Milton A. Reder practices at 28 Manchester Boulevard, Brookline, MA 02146. His telephone number is (617) 738-4279. Young Dr. Reder is one of the leading experts on the subject of the SGB. We have already written extensively about his background, so we will not repeat it here.

HERSCHEL L. STROUD, D.D.S.

Dr. Stroud practices dentistry at 1271 Woodhole, Topeka, KS 66604. His telephone number is (913) 273-4770. If you ask, Dr. Stroud will gladly tell you the story of how he became a practitioner of SGB.

One of his patients had been suffering from low back pain and sciatica for several months. The man was the CEO of a national chain of shoe stores and it was important for him to travel frequently and to be physically very active. However, pain had almost incapacitated him. He tried every possible treatment, and then one day a division manager told him about Dr. Reder. He went to New York to visit Reder and after three weeks of treatment his pain disappeared and he was able to resume all his activities. When he returned to Topeka, he tried unsuccessfully to induce some physician to perform the SGB. Finally, he told his dentist, Dr. Stroud, about his problem.

Dr. Stroud, although skeptical, agreed to visit Dr. Reder in New York. Dr. Stroud spent several days interviewing four hundred patients in Dr. Reder's office, and says he was "frankly amazed and impressed with the apparent clinical results." Just as I did, he also spent a day in the New York Academy of Medicine Library, researching the historical and medical background of SGB.

On returning to Topeka, he consulted with several physicians he knew at the Menninger Foundation, who urged him to try to duplicate the procedure in Topeka. At their suggestion, he did, and he presently administers the SGB himself in his office.

HAROLD C. WALRAVEN, D.D.S.

Dr. Walraven practices at 1957 Howell Mill Road, Atlanta, GA 30318. His telephone number is (404) 355-6770. Dr. Walraven was trained by Dr. Stroud. He specializes in the relief of pain in the head and neck. He has given successful demonstrations of the efficacy of the SGB before pain societies.

THE LEADING EXPERT IN THE FIELD

Asa P. Ruskin, M.D., F.A.C.P., is unquestionably the leading academician and expert in the field of the sphenopalatine ganglion blockade. He has not authorized me to put his name in this listing as a practitioner in the field. I know from others that his unit at the medical center, as well as Dr. Ruskin himself, does use the blockade on occasion. However, he treats it as one of the procedures among many which he uses in treatment.

Dr. Ruskin is the son of the famed Simon Ruskin, M.D., who in 1925 became the first physician to realize the full potential of the SGB. The latter Dr. Ruskin wrote extensively in the field and in modern times the work on the theory and application of the SGB has been carried on by his son, Dr. Asa P. Ruskin.

Dr. Asa P. Ruskin is the Director of Rehabilitation Medicine at the Kingsbrook Jewish Medical Center at 585 Schenectady Avenue, Brooklyn, NY 11203. The telephone number of the Center is (718) 604-5341. Dr. Ruskin is also Associate Clinical

Professor of Rehabilitation Medicine at the Albert Einstein College of Medicine in New York.

In addition to many articles in the medical journals on the various aspects of the SGB, Dr. Ruskin has edited a book entitled, *Current Therapy and Physiatry* (Philadelphia: Saunders, 1984). Dr. Ruskin, in addition to editing the book, wrote Chapter 7, entitled, "Treatment of Pain, Spasm, and Psychosomatic Symptoms Mediated Through the Sympathetic System, Including Sphenopalatine (Nasal) Ganglion Blockade."

That chapter will be of particular interest to physicians, biologists, and scientists because it offers a complete medical theory on what makes the blockade work and also describes in detail the techniques for performing the block.

Ruskin's chapter offers an important conclusion: "In my experience of 25 years, and the experience of Simon Ruskin extending for 40 years prior to that time, there have been no serious incidents of idiosyncratic reaction to the use of cocaine or other topical anesthesia."

APPENDIX II

Sphenopalatine Ganglion Block Bibliography

1893

Walker, A. Stodart. "A Case of Epileptiform Neuralgia—Excision of Meckel's Ganglion—Cure," *Edinb. Hosp. Rep.*, Vol 1: 416–419: 1893.

1909

Sluder, Greenfield. "The Anatomical and Clinical Relations of the Sphenopalatine (Meckel's) Ganglion to the Nose and Its Accessory Sinuses," *New York Med. J.*, Vol 90: 293–298: 1909.

1910

Sluder, Greenfield. "Further Clinical Observations on the Sphenopalatine Ganglion (Motor, Sensor, and Gustatory)," *Bulletin of the St. Louis Medical Society*, Vol 4: 64–65: 1910.

Sluder, Greenfield. "The Syndrome of Sphenopalatine Ganglion Neurosis," *Am. J. of Med. Science*, Vol 3: 868–878: 1910.

1916

Pollock, Harry L. "Difficulties and Complications of Sphenopalatine Ganglion Injection," *Annals of Oto., Rhin., and Laryng.*, Vol 25: 958–966, 1089–1096: 1916.

1921

Frazier, Charles H. "A Surgical Approach to the Sphenopalatine Ganglion," *Annals of Surg.*, Vol 74: 328–330: 1921.

1925

Ruskin, Simon L. "Herpes Zoster Oticus Relieved by Sphenopalatine Ganglion Treatment," *Laryngoscope*, Vol 35: 301–302: 1925.

Ruskin, Simon L. "The Surgical Aspect of the Nasal Ganglion," *N.Y. State J. of Med.*, Vol 25: 929–932: 1925.

Ruskin, Simon L. "Contributions to the Study of the Sphenopalatine Ganglion," *Laryngoscope*, Vol 35(2): 87–108: Feb. 1925.

1927

Chase, Walter D. "Sphenopalatine Ganglion Treatment of Certain Nose Conditions," *Atlantic Medical Journal*, Vol 0.30: 779–780: 1927.

Meyersburg, Harry. "Influence of Filtered Quartz Light on the Nasal Ganglion," *Arch. of Otolaryngol.*, Vol 5: 415–423: 1927.

Sluder, G. *Nasal Neurology, Headaches and Eye Disorders*, St. Louis, C. V. Mosby, 1927.

1928

Byrd, Hiram. "The Nasal Ganglion or Switchboard Test," *Medical Journal and Record*, Vol 128:68–71: 1928.

Gundrum, Lawrence K. "Migraine Controlled Through the Nasal Ganglion," *Arch. of Otolaryngology*, Vol 8:564–566: 1928.

Homme, O. H. "The Roentgen Ray as an Aid in the Injection of the Sphenopalatine Ganglion," *Arch. of Otolaryngol.*, Vol 7(6): 553–564: 1928.

1929

Dock, George. "Sluder's Nasal Ganglion Syndrome and Its Relation to Internal Medicine," *J. of the Am. Med. Assoc.*, Vol 93(10):750–753: Sept. 7, 1929.

Ruskin, Simon L. "The Neurologic Aspects of Nasal Sinus Infections," *Arch. of Otolaryngol.*, Vol 10(4):337–383: 1929.

1930
Byrd, Hiram. "The Sphenopalatine Test," *J. of Mich. Med. Soc*, Vol 29: 294–298: 1930.

Byrd, Hiram; Byrd, Wallace. "Sphenopalatine Phenomena—Present Status of Knowledge," *Arch. of Int. Med.*, Vol 46: 1026–1038: 1930.

Steward D.; Lambert, Victor. "Sphenopalatine Ganglion," *J. of Laryngol. and Otolaryngol.*, Vol 45:753–771: 1930.

1931
Van Osdol, H. A. "The Systemic Effect of Nasal Hyperplasia as it Affects the Nasal Ganglion," *J. Indiana Med. Assoc.*, Vol 24:3–8: 1931.

1934
Stewart D.; Lambert, Victor. "Further Observations on the Sphenopalatine Ganglion," *J. of Laryngol. and Otolaryn.* Vol 49: 319–323: 1934.

1935
Sparer, W. "Cessation of Convulsive Seizures Following Injection of Alcohol into the Sphenopalatine Ganglion in Three Cases," *Laryngoscope*. Vol 45:886–890: 1935.

1937
Dubois-Paulsen. "Le Ganglion Sphenopalatin et L'oeil," *Annals d'Occulistique*, Vol 174:217–248: 1937.

1938
Fenton, Ralph A. "Pathways of Referred Pain from the Nose," *Am. J. of Surg.*, Vol 42: 194–198: 1938.

1940
Rosen, Samuel; Shelesnyak, M. C.; Zacharias, L. R. "Naso-

genital Relationship. II Pseudo-pregnancy Following Extirpation of the Sphenopalatine Ganglion in the Rat," *Endocrinology,* Vol 27:463–468: 1940.

1941

Leudde, W. H. "The Relation of Meckel's Ganglion to Accommodation and Intraocular Tension," *Illinois Medical Journal,* Vol 79:199–209: 1941.

1942

Girling, Moray. "Lower Half Headache, Symptoms and Treatment," *Northwest Medicine,* Vol 41:418–419: 1942.

Gottesfeld, Ben H.; Leavitt, Frederic H. "Crocodile Tears, Treated by Injection into the Sphenopalatine Ganglion," *Arch. of Neurol. and Psychiatry,* Vol 47:314–315: 1942.

Hinsey, Joseph C.; Geohegan, William A.; Aidar, Orlando J. "Functional Reorganization of Sympathetic Ganglia Following Preganglionectomy," *Trans. of the Am. Neurol. Assoc.,* Vol 68:45–48: 1942.

Martin, Robert C. "Atypical Facial Neurologia," *Arch. of Otolaryngology,* Vol 35:735–739: 1942.

Ruskin, Simon. "Technique of Sphenopalatine Ganglion Therapy for Chorioretinitis," *Eye, Ear, Nose, and Throat Monthly,* Vol 30:735–739: 1942.

1944

Dysart, B. R. "Modern View of Neuralgia Referrable to Meckel's Ganglion," *Arch. of Otolaryngol.,* Vol 40:29–32: 1944.

Evans, Thomas H. "Nerve Branch at Superior Orbital Fissure Connecting Sixth Cranial with Component of Sphenopalatine Ganglion," *Am. J. of Ophthal.,* Vol 27:645–646: 1944.

1946

Ruskin, Simon L. "The Control of Muscle Spasm and Arthritic Pain Through Sympathetic Block at the Nasal Ganglion and the

Use of the Adenylic Nucleotide," *Am. J. of Digestive Diseases,* Vol 13(4):311–320: Apr. 1946.

Southworth, J. L. (Ed.). *Pitkin's Conduction Anesthesia,* Philadelphia, Lippincott (29–33, 82, 338–339, 356–357), 1946.

1948

Amster, J. Lewis. "Sphenopalatine Ganglion Block for the Relief of Painful Vascular and Muscular Spasm with Special Reference to Lumbro-Sacral Pain," *N.Y. State Med. J.,* Vol 48:2475–2480: 1948.

Laskiewicz, A. "Neurological Syndromes of Nasal Origin," *Acta Laryngscope,* Vol 36:203–219: 1948.

Wolff, H. G. "Cephalagias, and Atypical Neuralgias of the Face and Head," *Headaches and Other Head Pain,* New York, Oxford Univ. Press (411–429), 1948.

1949

Higbee, David. "Functional and Anatomic Relation of Sphenopalatine Ganglion to the Autonomic Nervous System," *Arch. of Otolaryngol.,* Vol 50:45–58: 1949.

Ruskin, Simon L. "A Newer Concept of Arthritis and the Treatment of Arthritic Pain and Deformity by Sympathetic Block at the Sphenopalatine (Nasal) Ganglion," *Am. J. of Digestive Diseases,* Vol 16:386–401: 1949.

1950

Poe, David L. "Transantral Approach for Excision of Sphenopalatine Ganglion for Intractable Facial Pain," *Arch. of Otolaryngol.,* Vol 51:891–900: 1950.

1951

Lewy, Robert B. "Anatomical and Clinical Evaluation of Head Pain Attributed to the Sphenopalatine Ganglion," *J. of Laryngol. and Otolaryng.,* Vol 65:10–13: 1951.

Ruskin, S. L. "Technic of Sphenopalatine Ganglion Therapy," *Eye, Ear, Nose, Throat Monthly,* Vol 30:28–31: 1951.

Sphenopalatine Ganglion Block Bibliography

1952

Rawlings, Maurice S.; Wise, Charles S. "Sphenopalatine Block in the Relief of Musculoskeletal Pain," *Arch. of Phy. Med.*, Vol 33:5–9: 1952.

1955

Hess, Arthur. "The Fine Structure of Young and Old Spinal Ganglia," *Anatomical Record,* Vol 123:399–412: 1955.

White, J. C. *Pain, Control and Mechanisms,* Springfield, Charles C. Thomas, 1955.

1959

Friedman, A. P. *Headache; Diagnosis and Treatment,* Philadelphia, F. A. Davis (102–103, 335–337), 1959.

1960

Langham, M. E.; Taylor, C. B. "The Influence of Superior Cervical Ganglionectomy on Intraocular Dynamics," *J. of Physiology,* Vol 152:447–458: 1960.

1968

Aubry, M.; Pialoux, P. "Sluder's Syndrome," *Handbook of Clinical Neurology: Vol 5, Headaches and Cranial Neurolgias,* Amsterdam, North-Holland Publishing Co. (326–332), 1968.

Bonica, J. "Autonomic Innervation and Nerve Block," *Anesthesiology*. Vol 29:793–813: 1968.

Haugen, J. "Autonomic Nervous System," *Anesthesiology,* Vol 29:785–792: 1968.

1970

Garlin, R. J. *Thomas' Oral Pathology*. Vol 2, 6th Ed, St. Louis, C. V. Mosby, 1096–1097: 1970.

Meyer, John S.; Binns, Philip M.; Ericsson, Arthur D.;e Vulpe, Michael. "Sphenopalatine Ganglionectomy for Cluster Headache," *Arch. of Otolaryng.*, Vol 92(5):475–484: Nov. 1970.

Sphenopalatine Ganglion Block Bibliography

1974

Gross, D. "International Symposium on Pain, Seattle, Wash.," *Adv. Neurology,* Vol 1: 4:93: 1974.

Procaci, P.; Francini, F.; et al. "Cutaneous Pain Threshold Changes After Sympathetic Block," *Pain,* Vol 1:167–175: 1975.

1975

1977

Ballenger, J. J. *Diseases of the Nose, Throat and Ear,* 12th Ed., Philadelphia, Lea and Febiger (10–11), 1977.

1979

Brown, Thomas W.; Sotereanos, George C. "Vascular Changes in the Pterygopalatine Fossa After Craniofacial Dysfunction Surgery," *J. of Oral. Surg,* Vol 37(2):88–92: Feb. 1979.

Gill, Claire J.; Orr II, Daniel L. "A Double-Blind Crossover Comparison of Topical Anesthetics," *J. Am. Dental Assoc.,* Vol 98(2):213–214: Feb 1979.

Graziussi, G.; Avella, F., Cacace, R.; Bracale, C.; Longhi, P. "Pizotifene Treatment of Sluder's Syndrome," *Acta Neurol.* (Napoli), Vol 34(1):73–75: Feb. 1979.

Hanowell, Susan T.; Kennedy, Stephen F. "Phantom Tongue Pain and Causalgia: Case Presentation and Treatment," *Anesthesia and Analgesia,* Vol 58(5):436–438: Sept.–Oct. 1979.

Jatlow, Peter; Barash, Paul G.; Van Dyke, Craig; Radding, Joel; Byck, Robert. "Cocaine and Succinylcholine Sensitivity: A New Caution," *Anesthesia and Analgesia,* Vol 58(3):235–238: May–Jun. 1979.

Manahan, A. P.; Orr, Roy. "Sphenopalatine Ganglion Block: An Effective Technique in the Management of Neck, Shoulder and Low Back Pain," written but unpublished, personal communication from author, Physical Medicine & Rehabilitation, Immanuel Medical Center, Omaha, Nebraska: 1979.

Mercuri, Louis G. "Intraoral Second Division Nerve Block," *J. of Oral Surg.*, Vol 37(9):109–113: Feb. 1979.

Panje, William R. "Local Anesthesia of the Face," *J. Dermatol Surg. Oncol.*, Vol 5(4):311–315: Apr. 1979.

Procacci, Paolo; Francini, Fabio; Maresca, Marco; Zoppi, Massimo. "Skin Potential and EMG Changes Induced by Cutaneous Electrical Stimulation," *Applied Neurophysiology*, Vol 42(3):125–134:1979.

Ruskin, Asa P. "Sphenopalatine (Nasal) Ganglion: Its Role in Pain, Spasm and the Rage Reaction and Possible Relationship to Acupuncture," *Int. J. Acupuncture and Electro-Therapeutics*, Vol 4: 91–103: 1979.

Ruskin, Asa P. "Sphenopalatine (Nasal) Ganglion: Remote Effects Including Psychosomatic Symptoms, Race Reaction, Pain, and Spasm," *Arch of Physical Medicine and Rehabilitation*, Vol 60(8):353–359: Aug. 1979.

Ryan, Robert E., Sr.; Ryan, Robert E. Jr. "Headaches of Nasal Origin," *Headache*, 173–177: Apr. 1979.

1980

Jordan, Alan; Baum, Jules. "Basic Tear Flow—Does It Exist?" *Amer. Academy of Opthalmology*, Vol 87(9): 920–930: Sep. 1980.

Khoury, Riad; Kennedy, Stephen F.; MacNamara, Thomas E. "Facial Causalgia: Report of Case," *J. of Oral Surg.*, Vol 38(10):782–783: Oct. 1980.

Lazar, Martin L.; Greenlee, Ralph G., Jr.; Naarden, Allan L. "Facial Pain of Neurologic Origin Mimicking Oral Pathologic Conditions: Some Current Concepts and Treatment," *J. of Am. Dent. Assoc.*, Vol 100:884–888: June 1980.

Osborn, Anne G. "The Vidian Artery—Normal and Pathologic Anatomy," *Radiology*, Vol 136(2):373–378: Aug. 1980.

Pryor, Gary J.; Kilpatrick, William R.; Opp, Duane R. "Local

Anesthesia in Minor Lacerations: Topical TAC vs. Lidocaine Infiltration," *Annals Emerg. Med.*, Vol 9(11):568:571: Nov. 1980.

Read, J. M.; Bach, P. H. "Sterile Topical Lignocaine Jelly in Plastic Surgery—An Assessment of its Systemic Toxicity," *Sa. Fr. Med. J.*, Vol 57(17):704–706: Apr. 1980.

Russo, Jr., John; Lipman, Arthur G.; Comstock, Thomas J.; Page, Brent C.; Stephen, Robert L. "Lidocaine Anesthesia: Comparison of Iontophoresis, Injection, and Swabbing," *Am. J. Hosp. Pharm.*, Vol 37(6):843–847: June 1980.

Sandza, Jr., Joseph G.; Roberts, Raymond W.; Shaw, Richard C.; Connors, John P. "Symptomatic Methemoglobinemia with a Commonly Used Topical Anesthetic, Cetacaine," *Annals Thorac, Surg.*, Vol 30(2):187–190: Aug. 1980.

Turvey, Timothy A.; Fonseca, Raymond J. "The Anatomy of the Internal Maxillary Artery in the Pterygopalatine Fossa: Its Relationship to Maxillary Surgery," *J. of Oral Surgery*, Vol 38(2):92–95: Feb. 1980.

1981

Kunkel, R. S. "A Complexity of Headaches," *Emergency Medicine*, Vol 13:24:1981.

Lukomsky, G. I.; Ovchinnikov, A. A.; Bilal, Ahmed. "Complications of Bronchoscopy—Comparison of Rigid Bronchoscopy Under General Anesthesia and Flexible Fiberoptic Bronchoscopy Under Topical Anesthesia," *Chest*, Vol 79(3):316–321: Mar. 1981.

1982

Yang, J. C.; Clark, W. C.; et al. "Effect of Intranasal Cocaine on Experimental Pain in Man," *Anesthesiology and Analgesia*, Vol 61:358–361: 1982.

1983

Klein, R. S. "Sphenopalatine Ganglion Block in Chronic Pain,"

Abstracts: World Congress on Scientific Acupuncture, Vienna, Austria: Oct. 1983.

1984

Klein, R. S. "Efficacy of Sphenopalatine Ganglion Block in the Treatment of Acute and Chronic Pain," in Supplement No. 2, Fourth World Congress on Pain, Seattle, Wash., 1984.

Ruskin, A. P. "Treatment of Pain, Spasm, and Psychosomatic Symptoms Mediated Through the Sympathetic System, Including Sphenopalatine (Nasal) Ganglion Blockade," in *Current Therapy in Physiatry*, Philadelphia, Saunders, 1984.

APPENDIX III

From Supplement No. 2, Fourth World Congress on Pain, in Seattle, Washington, 1984, held by the International Association for the Study of Pain.

EFFICACY OF SPHENOPALATINE GANGLION (SPG) BLOCK IN THE TREATMENT OF ACUTE AND CHRONIC PAIN. R. S. Klein, Dept.[*] of Medicine, N.Y. Medical College, N.Y., USA.

Aim of Investigation: The Autonomic Nervous System has been accepted as intimately involved in many acute and chronic pain syndromes. Interruption of transmission of sympathetic conduction to the periphery, either by injectable anesthetic or by permanent surgical intervention, is an accepted mainstay to our approach to alleviating these pain syndromes.

SPG block has been well described and is an accepted method of treating various cranio-facial pain syndromes, such as cluster headaches and trigeminal neuralgia. At the beginning of this century, many reports suggested that blocking the SPG by various methods could effect alleviation of pain syndromes at a distance from the ganglion (and apparently anatomically unrelated), among them, sciatica, bursitis, osteoarthritis, cancer pain and a host of others. This study examines the efficacy of the SPG block and its usefulness in pain management.

Methods: 2,000 patients with various acute and chronic pain syndromes, i.e., cancer, arthritis, discogenic disease, etc., were treated with SPG block. Four flexible Q-tips were inserted through the nasal passages to rest upon the SPG area. Each Q-tip has one drop of a 25% cocaine solution.

Results: 70.2% of various vascular musculo-skeletal pain syndromes became pain-free following daily blocks. Treatment required daily blocks (ranging from 1-14 days). Another 17.8% of patients were markedly improved but required weekly follow-up treatments to maintain a pain-free or pain-diminished status. Pain alleviation of cancer patients was equally impressive.

Conclusions: The superficial location of the SPG is innocuous, non-invasive and safe, with virtually no side effects. SPG block is an impressive and effective additional tool in pain management without the associated side effects of drugs. Importantly, the quality of life is enhanced in these patients.

About the Author

Albert B. Gerber is a well-known Philadelphia lawyer and a published author. He has written seven books on a variety of subjects, as well as numerous articles and fiction in popular magazines. His learned articles have appeared in major Law Review periodicals.

Albert Gerber is well qualified to do research on almost any topic. He holds the degrees of B.S. in Ed., M.A. in Gov., LL.M. and J.D. from several major American universities.

The author has first-hand knowledge of the procedure described herein. He suffered from severe back pain which the medical experts could neither explain nor relieve. When he heard about Dr. Milton Reder, he went to Park Avenue looking for relief from pain, and he stayed to do the research needed to share with others what he found.